RECOMMENDED COMMUNITY STRATEGIES AND MEASUREMENTS TO PREVENT OBESITY IN THE UNITED STATES:

Implementation and Measurement Guide

July 2009

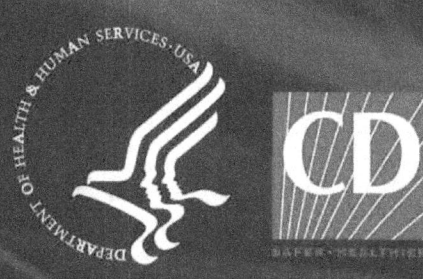

Acknowledgments

This guide was written by Dana Keener, PhD[1]; Kenneth Goodman, MA[1]; Amy Lowry, MPA[2]; Susan Zaro, MPH[1]; and Laura Kettel Khan, PhD.[3] All members of the Project Work Groups who contributed to this project are listed in Appendix A. ICF Macro served as the coordinating center for this project. Support for this project was provided to the CDC Foundation by the Robert Wood Johnson Foundation, the W.K. Kellogg Foundation, and Kaiser Permanente.

[1] *ICF Macro*
[2] *CDC Foundation*
[3] *Centers for Disease Control and Prevention*

Recommended Citation:

Keener, D., Goodman, K., Lowry, A., Zaro, S., & Kettel Khan, L. (2009). *Recommended community strategies and measurements to prevent obesity in the United States: Implementation and measurement guide.* Atlanta, GA: U.S. Department of Health and Human Services, Centers for Disease Control and Prevention.

For more information or to download this document, please visit:

http://www.cdc.gov/NCCDPHP/DNPAO/Publications/index.html

Preface

CDC is pleased to release **Recommended Community Strategies and Measurements to Prevent Obesity in the United States: Implementation and Measurement Guide.** This product is the result of an innovative and collaborative process that seeks to reverse the U.S. obesity epidemic by transforming communities into places where healthy lifestyle choices are easily incorporated into everyday life. Where we live, work, learn, worship, and play affects the choices we make, and in turn, our health. As such, the policies and environments that shape and define a community will also affect the health outcomes of its citizens. For example, communities that enact policies which increase access to affordable healthy food options and safe opportunities for physical activity create an environment by which individuals may be more likely to adopt a healthy eating, active living lifestyle. Reversing the U.S. obesity epidemic will require population level change that focuses on adopting policies and creating environments that support healthier lifestyle choices.

TABLE OF CONTENTS

INTRODUCTION 1

CATEGORY 1: STRATEGIES TO PROMOTE THE AVAILABILITY OF AFFORDABLE HEALTHY FOOD AND BEVERAGES 7

CATEGORY 2: STRATEGIES TO SUPPORT HEALTHY FOOD AND BEVERAGE CHOICES 21

CATEGORY 3: STRATEGY TO ENCOURAGE BREASTFEEDING 31

CATEGORY 4: STRATEGIES TO ENCOURAGE PHYSICAL ACTIVITY OR LIMIT SEDENTARY ACTIVITY AMONG CHILDREN AND YOUTH 35

CATEGORY 5: STRATEGIES TO CREATE SAFE COMMUNITIES THAT SUPPORT PHYSICAL ACTIVITY 45

CATEGORY 6: STRATEGY TO ENCOURAGE COMMUNITIES TO ORGANIZE FOR CHANGE 63

REFERENCES 67

APPENDIX A: PROJECT WORK GROUPS 73

APPENDIX B: TERMS USED IN THIS MANUAL 77

APPENDIX C: USEFUL CONTACTS FOR DATA COLLECTION 83

INTRODUCTION

INTRODUCTION

Obesity in the United States

America has a serious weight problem. Two-thirds of adults and nearly one-fifth of children in the United States are overweight, placing them at greater risk for heart disease, diabetes, and other chronic diseases including cancer and arthritis (Ogden et al., 2006; Ogden, Carroll, & Flegal, 2008). Furthermore, obesity and its related health problems are placing a major strain on the U.S. health care system. Americans cannot afford to put on more pounds—we must turn this problem around.

Where People Live, Work, and Play Affects Their Health

Local policies and the physical environment influence daily choices that affect our health—and our weight (Bell & Rubin, 2007). For example, children who live in unsafe neighborhoods may be restricted to watching television indoors instead of playing outside after school. Families living in neighborhoods that are zoned exclusively for residential use must drive to work and school because it is too far to walk. Communities that lack full-service grocery stores and neighborhood food markets have less access to fresh fruits and vegetables. Moreover, policies that establish physical activity requirements and nutrition standards in schools and daycare facilities can promote the health and well-being of children. These are just a few examples of how policies and the environment can affect what we eat and how we move, which in turn affects our health.

To reverse the obesity epidemic, we must change our physical and food environments to provide more opportunities for people to eat healthy foods and to be physically active on a daily basis. Accordingly, this manual describes 24 recommended strategies by the Centers for Disease Control and Prevention (CDC) to encourage and support healthy eating and active living. In addition, a single measure is provided for each strategy to help communities track their progress over time.

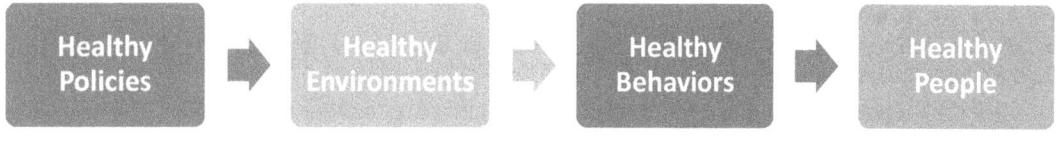

Local Governments' Role in Reversing the Obesity Epidemic

Many aspects of our physical environment that influence our health are created, managed, and maintained by local governments. For example, local policies and incentives can affect the presence and absence of parks, sidewalks, bike lanes, mixed-use development, healthy food retailers, and farmers markets. Public schools—although not under the authority of local governments—also have a vital role in ensuring that children have access to healthy food and sufficient opportunities for physical activity during the school day. Clearly, local governments and public school systems can make a real difference in creating healthy food and activity environments that benefit all people living in their communities.

Aside from the health benefits, there are also economic benefits to local governments for creating walkable, safe, and food-secure environments. For example, home values are expected to rise faster in "smart communities" that are made pedestrian-friendly by employing mixed-use development, sidewalks, and traffic-calming features (Local Government Commission Center for Livable Communities, n.d.).

How Local Governments Can Use Strategies and Measures of Environmental and Policy-Level Change

In order for local governments to target strategic investments that promote healthy eating and active living in their communities, they need information about the current conditions in their community that could be improved to better facilitate the health of their citizens. In addition, communities need tools to track their progress over time and to compare themselves to other similar communities on measures of environmental and policy change for obesity prevention. Accordingly, the 24 strategies and measures presented in this manual are designed to meet these needs. More specifically, the strategies and measures can be used by local governments and communities in three ways:

1. **For baseline assessment**
    - Do the policies and environmental conditions in our community currently promote active living and healthy eating?
    - How do our policies and environmental conditions compare to other communities of similar size, type, and population?

2. **To identify priorities for action**
    - What aspects of our environment are in greatest need of improvement to promote the health of our citizens?
    - Which strategies should we choose to implement to become a healthier community?

3. **To measure change over time**
    - Are we making progress from year to year in changing policies and environmental conditions to promote active living and healthy eating?

How the Strategies and Measures Were Identified and Developed

The strategies described in this manual are the product of an intensive collaborative process involving a cadre of nutrition and active living experts. A literature search was conducted to identify a broad range of environmental and policy-level strategies for obesity prevention. The results of the search were reviewed and narrowed by a select panel of nutrition and active living experts who were asked to prioritize the strategies based on their potential for extended reach, mutability, transferability, effectiveness, and sustainability.

After the strategies were identified, nutrition and active living experts and local government representatives were asked to nominate measures for each strategy while considering the criteria of utility, construct validity, and feasibility of each measure. Next, experts discussed the merits and limitations of each nominated measure during a series of teleconferences. Based on these discussions, experts selected a preferred measure for each strategy, which were then vetted by measurement experts and pilot tested by 20 local government representatives recruited by the Center for Performance Measurement of the International City/County Management Association. The measures were then further revised to ensure that they were feasible and useful to local governments. A complete description of the methodology used to identify and select the recommended strategies and measures is available at <http://www.cdc.gov/NCCDPHP/DNPAO/Publications/index.html>.

Limitations of the Strategies and Measures

The strategies and measures presented in this manual represent an early step in our understanding of how the environment and policies influence behavior. We are still accumulating evidence to support each strategy and the measures are not yet validated and their reliability has yet to be determined. The strategies do not represent an exhaustive list of the types of changes that need to occur and some may prove to be more important than others in relation to desired behavioral changes that affect health. Even with these limitations, these strategies and measures are an important starting point for addressing the obesity epidemic in the United States.

CDC's Recommended Strategies for Obesity Prevention

Communities should do the following:

1. Increase availability of healthier food and beverage choices in public service venues
2. Improve availability of affordable healthier food and beverage choices in public service venues
3. Improve geographic availability of supermarkets in underserved areas
4. Provide incentives to food retailers to locate in and/or offer healthier food and beverage choices in underserved areas
5. Improve availability of mechanisms for purchasing foods from farms
6. Provide incentives for the production, distribution, and procurement of foods from local farms
7. Restrict availability of less healthy foods and beverages in public service venues
8. Institute smaller portion size options in public service venues
9. Limit advertisements of less healthy foods and beverages
10. Discourage consumption of sugar-sweetened beverages
11. Increase support for breastfeeding
12. Require physical education in schools
13. Increase the amount of physical activity in physical education programs in schools
14. Increase opportunities for extracurricular physical activity
15. Reduce screen time in public service venues
16. Improve access to outdoor recreational facilities
17. Enhance infrastructure supporting bicycling
18. Enhance infrastructure supporting walking
19. Support locating schools within easy walking distance of residential areas
20. Improve access to public transportation
21. Zone for mixed-use development
22. Enhance personal safety in areas where persons are or could be physically active
23. Enhance traffic safety in areas where persons are or could be physically active
24. Participate in community coalitions or partnerships to address obesity

Using This Guide

The 24 strategies and measures presented in this manual are divided into 6 categories that represent different aspects of the physical and food environments. Each strategy is paired with one measure and is presented as follows:

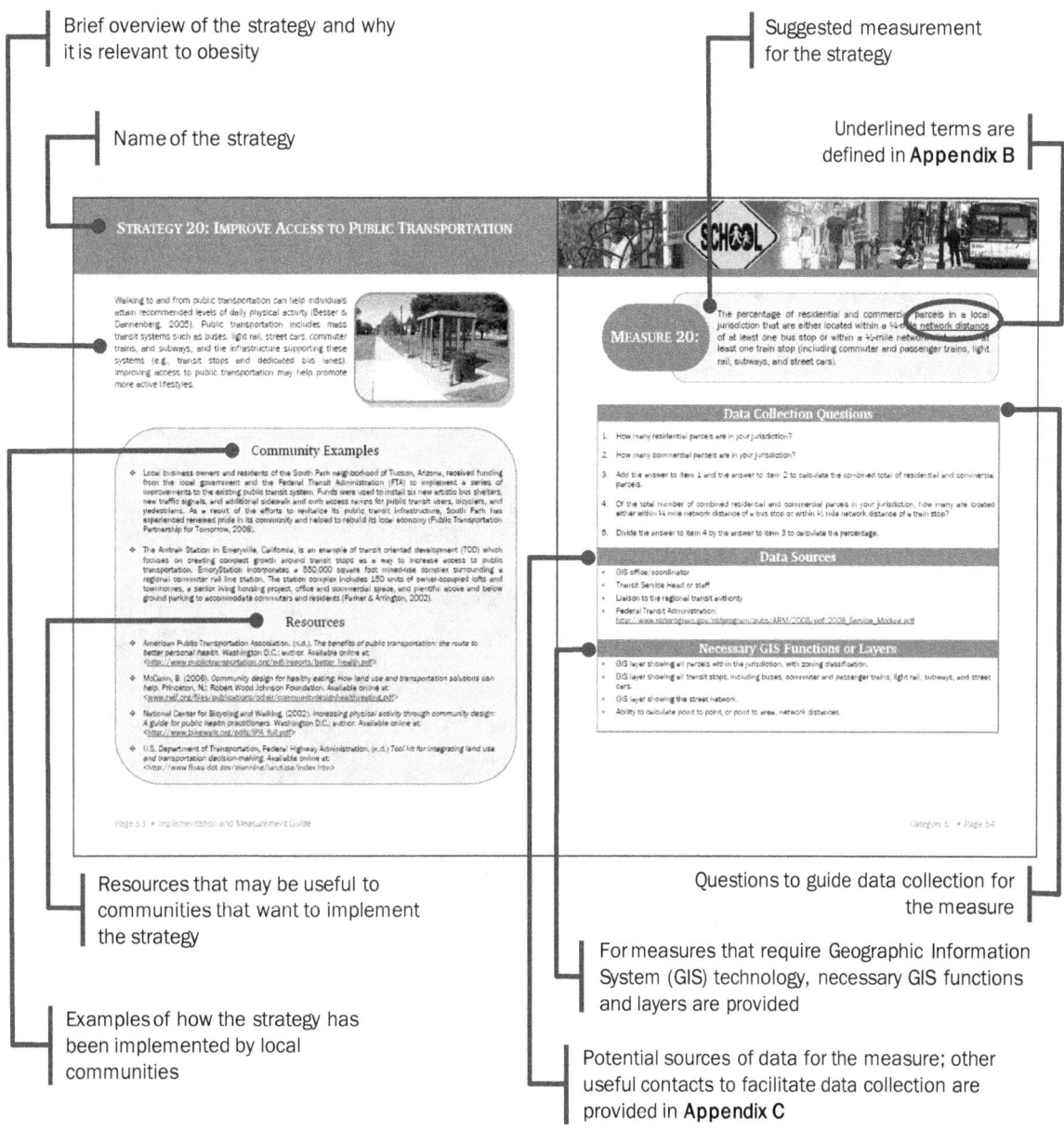

Brief overview of the strategy and why it is relevant to obesity

Name of the strategy

Suggested measurement for the strategy

Underlined terms are defined in **Appendix B**

Resources that may be useful to communities that want to implement the strategy

Examples of how the strategy has been implemented by local communities

Questions to guide data collection for the measure

For measures that require Geographic Information System (GIS) technology, necessary GIS functions and layers are provided

Potential sources of data for the measure; other useful contacts to facilitate data collection are provided in **Appendix C**

CATEGORY 1:
STRATEGIES TO PROMOTE THE AVAILABILITY OF AFFORDABLE HEALTHY FOOD AND BEVERAGES

STRATEGY 1: INCREASE AVAILABILITY OF HEALTHIER FOOD AND BEVERAGE CHOICES IN PUBLIC SERVICE VENUES

Limited availability of healthier food and beverage choices (e.g., foods with low calorie, sugar, fat, and sodium content) can be a barrier to healthy eating and drinking. Public service venues, such as schools, child care centers, city and county buildings, prisons, and juvenile detention centers, are key venues for increasing the availability of healthier foods. Improving the availability of healthier food and beverage choices (e.g., fruits, vegetables, and water) may increase the consumption of healthier foods.

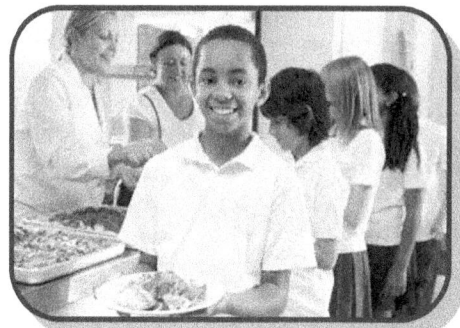

Community Examples

- In St. Paul, Minnesota, the "Five a Day Power Plus Program" increased the variety of fruits and vegetables offered in schools by providing an additional fruit item on days baked desserts were served, promoting fruits and vegetables at point-of-purchase, and enhancing the attractiveness of fruits and vegetables. Evaluation of the program found that fruit and vegetable consumption increased significantly among children in the intervention group as compared with a control group (Perry et al., 1998).

- In 2008, New York City became the first major city in the United States to set nutrition standards for all foods sold or served in city agencies, including schools, senior centers, homeless shelters, child care centers, afterschool programs, correctional facilities, public hospitals, and parks. The standards require city agencies to include two servings of fruits and vegetables in every lunch and dinner, phase out deep frying, lower salt content, serve healthier beverages, and increase the amount of fiber in meals (New York City Mayor's Office, 2008).

Resources

- Joint Center for Political and Economic Studies. (2004). *A place for healthier living: Improving access to physical activity and healthy foods.* Washington, DC: Author. Available online at: <http://www.policylink.org/pdfs/JointCenter-Healthyliving.pdf>

- Leadership for Healthy Communities. (2007). *Improving access to healthy foods: A guide for policy-makers.* Washington, DC: Robert Wood Johnson Foundation. Available online at: <http://www.leadershipforhealthycommunities.org/images/stories/healthyeatingweb.pdf>

- U.S. Department of Agriculture. (2005). *Making it happen! School nutrition success stories.* Alexandria, VA: Author. Available online at: <http://www.fns.usda.gov/TN/Resources/makingithappen.html>

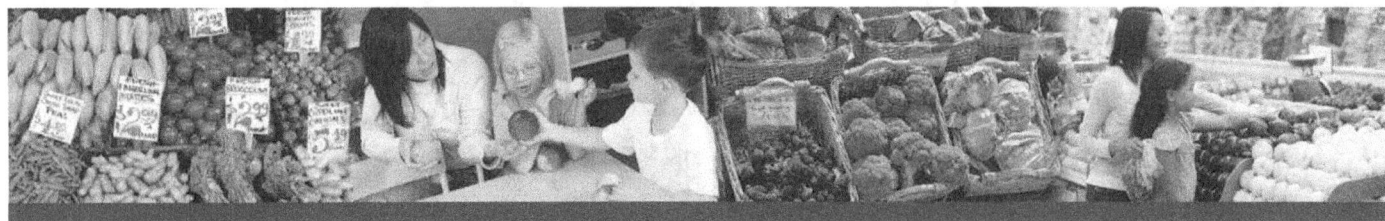

MEASURE 1: A policy exists to apply <u>nutrition standards</u>* that are consistent with the Dietary Guidelines for Americans to all food sold (e.g., meal menus and vending machines) within <u>local government facilities</u> in a local jurisdiction or on public school campuses during the school day within the <u>largest school district in a local jurisdiction</u>.

* All underlined terms are defined in Appendix B for the purpose of measurement.

Data Collection Questions

1. Does your local government have a policy to apply nutrition standards that are consistent with the Dietary Guidelines for Americans to all food sold (e.g., foods sold in cafeterias and vending machines) within local government facilities?

    1a. If you answered yes to question 1, to which of the following types of local government facilities does the policy apply?

    - Administrative office facilities
    - 24-hour "dormitory-type" facilities
    - Health care facilities
    - Recreation/community center facilities
    - Detention facilities
    - Other facilities

    1b. If you answered yes to question 1, please describe the nutrition standards.

    1c. Is there a State policy or requirement regarding nutrition standards that applies to your local jurisdiction?

2. Does the largest school district within your local jurisdiction have a policy to apply nutrition standards that are consistent with the Dietary Guidelines for Americans to all food sold (e.g., foods sold in cafeterias and vending machines) on public school campuses during the school day?

    2a. If you answered yes to question 2, please describe the nutrition standards.

Data Sources

- Office that maintains government-wide policies (e.g., city/county manager's office, mayor's office)
- Department of Facilities Management
- Purchasing staff person who manages the food service or vending contract for jurisdiction
- School district's administrative office, such as the district school food authority

STRATEGY 2: IMPROVE AVAILABILITY OF AFFORDABLE HEALTHIER FOOD AND BEVERAGE CHOICES IN PUBLIC SERVICE VENUES

Healthier foods are generally more expensive than less healthy foods, posing an economic barrier to healthier eating, particularly among low-income populations (Drewnowski, 2004). Public schools and local governments can improve the affordability of healthier foods and beverages sold in public service venues by establishing policies that lower prices of healthier foods and beverages relative to the cost of less healthy foods sold in vending machines, cafeterias, and concession stands in schools and local government facilities. Other strategies to make healthy food more affordable include offering coupons or vouchers redeemable for healthier foods and incentives or bonuses for the purchase of healthier foods.

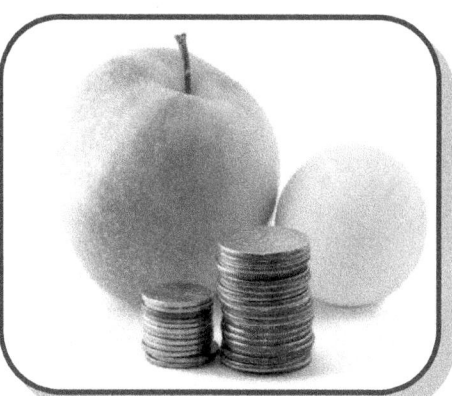

Community Examples

❖ The New York City Department of Health operates the Health Bucks Program to make fruits and vegetables more affordable to residents who receive food stamps. For every five dollars' worth of food stamps spent at farmers' markets, individuals receive a $2 Health Bucks coupon which can be redeemed year round at more than 30 farmers' markets citywide. In 2007, the City Health Department reported that New Yorkers used more than 40% of the 9,000 Health Bucks distributed in 2006 (New York City Department of Health and Mental Hygiene, 2007).

❖ In 2004, the Seattle School Board unanimously approved nutrition-related policies designed to provide healthy and affordable food and beverage options to students. As a result, all campus vending machines and student stores are now required to sell beverages such as soda, juice, and sports drinks at a higher price than bottled water. The policy was implemented in all elementary, middle, and high schools throughout the Seattle School District (Seattle Public Schools, 2004).

Resources

❖ California Project LEAN and the Center for Weight and Health. (2006). *Policy in action: A guide to implementing your local school wellness policy.* Sacramento: California Project LEAN. Available online at: <http://www.californiaprojectlean.org/Assets/1019/files/Policy%20in%20Action%20Guide%20FINAL.pdf>

❖ Flourney, R., & Treuhaft, S. (2005). *Healthy food, healthy communities: Improving access and opportunities through food retailing.* Oakland, CA: PolicyLink. Available online at: <http://www.policylink.org/pdfs/HealthyFoodHealthyCommunities.pdf>

❖ U.S. Department of Agriculture. (2005). *Making it happen! School nutrition success stories.* Alexandria, VA: Author. Available online at: <http://www.fns.usda.gov/TN/Resources/makingithappen.html>

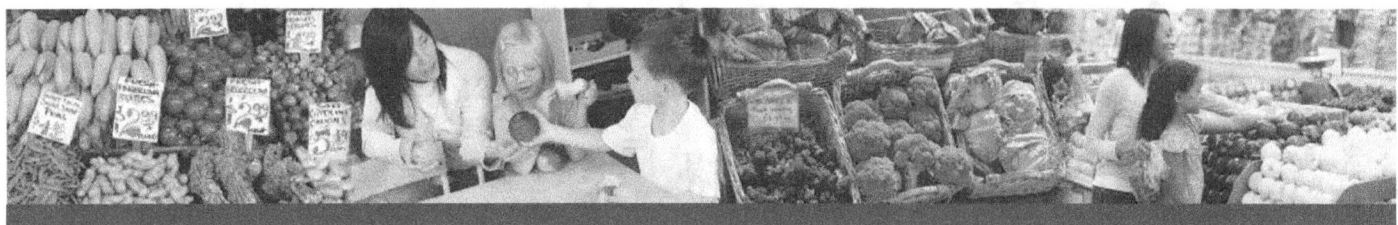

MEASURE 2:

A policy exists to affect the cost of <u>healthier foods and beverages</u> relative to the cost of <u>less healthy foods and beverages</u> sold within <u>local government facilities</u> in a local jurisdiction or on public school campuses during the school day within the <u>largest school district in a local jurisdiction</u>.

Data Collection Questions

1. Does your local government have a policy to affect the cost of healthier foods and beverages relative to the cost of less healthy foods and beverages sold in local government facilities?

   1a. If you answered yes to question 1, to which of the following types of foods does your local government's policy regarding pricing of healthier food apply?

   - Entrees/main courses/sandwiches
   - Dairy
   - Fruits
   - Vegetables
   - Beverages
   - Snacks
   - Other (please specify)

   1b. If you answered yes to question 1, to which of the following types of facilities does your local government's policy regarding pricing of healthier food apply?

   - Administrative office facilities
   - 24-hour "dormitory-type" facilities
   - Health care facilities
   - Recreation/community center facilities
   - Detention facilities
   - Other facilities

   1c. If you answered yes to question 1, please describe your local government's food pricing policy.

   1d. Is there a State policy or requirement regarding food pricing that applies to your local jurisdiction?

2. Does the largest school district within your local jurisdiction have a policy to affect the cost of healthier foods and beverages relative to the cost of less healthy foods and beverages sold on public school campuses during the school day within the district?

   2a. If you answered yes to question 2, to which of the following types of foods does your school district's policy regarding pricing of healthier food apply?

   - Entrees/main courses/sandwiches
   - Dairy
   - Fruits
   - Vegetables
   - Beverages
   - Snacks
   - Other (please specify)

   2b. If you answered yes to question 2, please describe the school district's food pricing policy.

Data Sources

- School district administrative offices
- Facilities managers and/or parks and recreation staff
- Local government office that maintains government policies

STRATEGY 3: IMPROVE GEOGRAPHIC AVAILABILITY OF SUPERMARKETS IN UNDERSERVED AREAS

Supermarkets have a larger selection of healthy food at lower prices compared to smaller grocery stores and convenience stores. However, research indicates that low-income, minority, and rural communities have fewer supermarkets as compared to more affluent areas (Larson, Story, & Nelson, 2008; Morland, Wing, Diez Roux, & Poole, 2002). Increasing the number of supermarkets in areas where they are currently unavailable or where availability is limited is one way to increase access to healthy foods, particularly for economically disadvantaged populations.

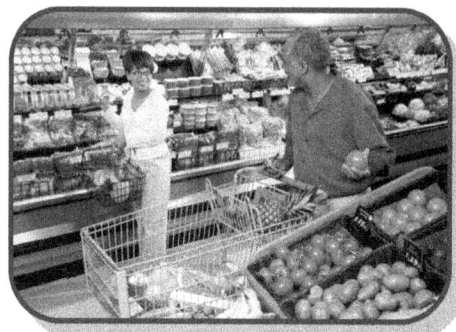

Community Examples

❖ The Philadelphia Food Marketing Task Force investigated the lack of supermarkets in Philadelphia and released 10 recommendations to increase the number of supermarkets in Philadelphia's underserved communities. A new funding initiative was created using public funds to leverage supermarket development. To date, the initiative has committed $67 million in funding for 69 supermarket projects in 27 Pennsylvania counties, creating or preserving 3,900 jobs (Burton & Duane, 2004).

❖ In Hartford, Connecticut, an Advisory Commission on Food Policy studied the local food system and launched an initiative to improve bus service routes to grocery stores and to reduce food prices in low-income areas. The commission created a special cross-town bus route that cut travel time in half for low-income residents to reach a shopping area with a major supermarket. A survey of the bus line riders found that one-third of the riders were using the bus route to reach the supermarkets (McCann, 2006).

Resources

❖ Leadership for Healthy Communities. (2007). *Improving access to healthy foods: A guide for policy-makers*. Washington, DC: Robert Wood Johnson Foundation. Available online at:
<http://www.rwjf.org/files/research/accesshealthyfoodslhc2007.pdf>

❖ McCann, B. (2006). *Community design for healthy eating: How land use and transportation solutions can help*. Princeton, NJ: Robert Wood Johnson Foundation. Available online at:
<http://www.rwjf.org/files/publications/other/communitydesignhealthyeating.pdf>

❖ PolicyLink and Bay Area LISC. (2007). *Grocery store attraction strategies: A resource for community activists and local governments*. Oakland, CA: Author. Available online at:
<http://www.policylink.org/mailings/publications/store_attraction.pdf>

❖ Strategic Alliance ENACT. (n.d.). *Attract supermarkets to underserved areas*. Retrieved April 13, 2009, from
<http://www.preventioninstitute.org/sa/enact/neighborhood/supermarkets_underserved.php>

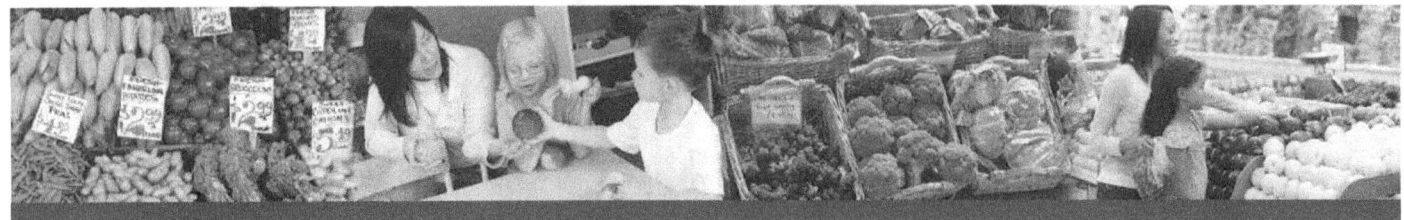

MEASURE 3: The number of <u>full-service grocery stores</u> and <u>supermarkets</u> per 10,000 residents located within the three largest <u>underserved census tracts</u> within a local jurisdiction.

Data Collection Questions

1. What is the total combined population of the three largest underserved census tracts within your local jurisdiction? Divide this number by 10,000.

2. What is the total number of full-service grocery stores and supermarkets located within the three largest underserved census tracts within your jurisdiction?

3. Divide the answer to question 2 by the answer to item 1.

Example:

1. 13,000 residents / 10,000 = 1.3
2. 2 full-service grocery stores
3. 2 / 1.3 = 1.54 grocery stores per 10,000 residents

Data Sources

- Business license office
- Geographic Information System (GIS) office/coordinator
- Chamber of Commerce

Necessary GIS Functions or Layers

- GIS layer showing the census tracts within the jurisdiction, including coding that shows specifically which tracts meet the definition of underserved
- Ability to determine population by census tract

STRATEGY 4: PROVIDE INCENTIVES TO FOOD RETAILERS TO LOCATE IN AND/OR OFFER HEALTHIER FOOD AND BEVERAGE CHOICES IN UNDERSERVED AREAS

Limited availability of healthier food and beverage choices in underserved communities poses a significant barrier to improving nutrition and preventing obesity (Morland, Wing, & Diez Roux, 2002). Local governments can offer financial and nonfinancial incentives to food retailers (e.g., grocery stores) to open new stores and/or to offer healthier food and beverage choices in areas with few healthy food options. Financial incentives include, but are not limited to, tax breaks, tax credits, loans, loan guarantees, and grants to cover start-up and investment costs. Nonfinancial incentives include supportive zoning, negotiation assistance, and capacity building for small businesses that want to initiate sales of healthier foods and beverages.

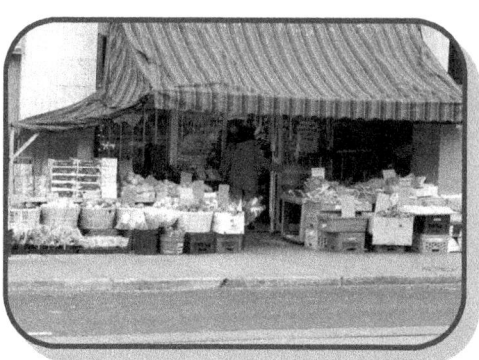

Community Examples

- The city of Richmond, California, attracted a national discount grocery store to an urban retail center with adjacent affordable housing by offering an attractive incentive package, which included land sold at a reduced cost to the developer; a Federal Urban Development Action Grant of $3.5 million for commercial development; a zoning designation that provided tax incentives; assistance in negotiations with State regulatory agencies; improvements to surrounding sidewalks, streetscape, and traffic signals; and concessions on design standards (PolicyLink & Bay Area Local Initiatives Support Corporation, 2008).

- New York City's FRESH Program provides zoning and financial incentives to property owners, developers, and grocery store operators in areas of the city currently underserved by grocery stores. Although other cities have restricted unhealthy food outlets or provided funding for supermarkets on individual sites, FRESH is the first program in the nation to combine zoning and financial incentives and to offer them in multiple neighborhoods. FRESH will help create an estimated 15 new grocery stores and upgrade 10 existing stores, creating 1,100 new jobs and retaining 400 others (City of New York, 2009).

Resources

- Flourney, R., & Treuhaft, S. (2005). *Healthy food, healthy communities: Improving access and opportunities through food retailing*. Oakland, CA: PolicyLink. Available online at:
  <http://www.policylink.org/pdfs/HealthyFoodHealthyCommunities.pdf>

- PolicyLink and Bay Area LISC. (2007). *Grocery store attraction strategies: A resource for community activists and local governments*. Oakland, CA: Authors. Available online at:
  <http://www.policylink.org/mailings/publications/store_attraction.pdf>

- PolicyLink. (n.d.). *Equitable development toolkit: Healthy food retailing*. Retrieved April 13, 2009, from:
  <http://www.policylink.org/EDTK/HealthyFoodRetailing/default.html>

- Strategic Alliance ENACT. (n.d.). *Provide training and incentives to small store owners underserved areas to carry healthier food items, such as fresh produce*. Retrieved April 13, 2009, from:
  <http://www.preventioninstitute.org/sa/enact/neighborhood/shopkeepers.php>

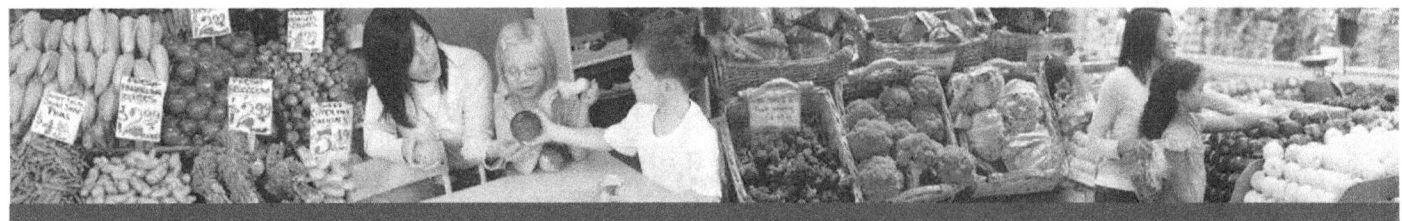

MEASURE 4:
Local government offers at least one incentive to new and/or existing food retailers to offer <u>healthier food and beverage choices</u> in underserved areas.

Data Collection Questions

1. Does your local government offer at least one incentive (financial or nonfinancial) to new and/or existing food retailers to offer healthier food and beverage choices in underserved areas?

    1a. If you answered yes to question 1, which of the following incentive(s) are offered to local retailers?
    - Tax benefits, tax credits, or tax breaks
    - Loans
    - Technical assistance/negotiation assistance
    - Waivers for local ordinance requirements
    - Other

Data Sources

- City/county manager's office
- Economic development office
- Chamber of Commerce

STRATEGY 5: IMPROVE AVAILABILITY OF MECHANISMS FOR PURCHASING FOODS FROM FARMS

Farmers markets, farm stands, community-supported agriculture (CSA), pick your own, and farm-to-school initiatives are all ways to purchase food from farms. Increasing the availability of such mechanisms for purchasing foods from farms may reduce costs of fresh foods through direct sales, increase the availability of fresh foods in areas without supermarkets, and improve the nutritional value and taste of fresh foods by harvesting produce at ripeness rather than at a time conducive to shipping (M. Hamm, personal communication, May 19, 2008).

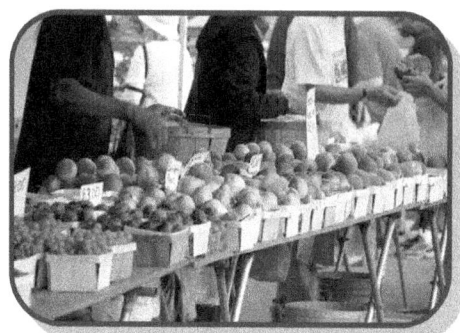

Community Examples

- In 2005, Jefferson Elementary School, in Riverside, California, launched a farm-to-school salad bar program which provides elementary school students access to a daily salad bar stocked with a variety of locally grown produce as an alternative to the standard hot lunch. Two small, locally owned family farms, within 30 miles of the school, sell their produce at an affordable price and make weekly deliveries to the school. Since implementing the farm-to-school salad bar program, the Riverside school district has expanded the program to four additional elementary schools (Anupama, Kalb, & Beery, 2006).

- The Food Trust's Farmers' Market Program operates a network of 30 farmers' markets serving more than 125,000 customers in the Philadelphia region of Pennsylvania. Many of the farmers' markets are located in neighborhoods underserved by supermarkets, grocery stores, and other fresh food outlets. All of the farmers' markets accept food stamps (EBT/Access cards) and Farmers' Market Nutrition Program vouchers. <http://www.thefoodtrust.org>

Resources

- Joshi, A., Kalb, M., & Berry, M. (2006). *Going local: Paths to success for farm to school programs.* Los Angeles, CA: National Farm to School Program Center for Food and Justice and Community Food Security Coalition. Available online at: <http://departments.oxy.edu/uepi/cfj/publications/goinglocal.pdf>

- Michigan Department of Community Health. (n.d.). *Healthy Communities tool kit: How you can work toward creating healthy communities.* Lansing, MI: Author. Available online at: <http://www.mihealthtools.org/documents/HealthyCommunitiesToolkit_web.pdf>

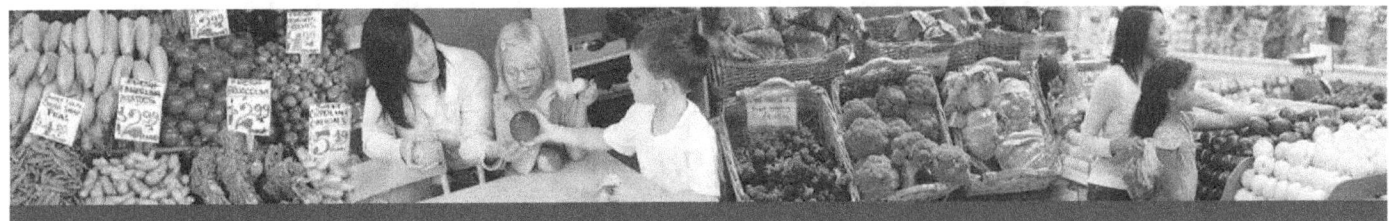

Measure 5:
The total annual number of <u>farmer-days</u> at <u>farmers markets</u> per 10,000 residents within a local jurisdiction.

Data Collection Questions

1. How many farmers markets operate within your local jurisdiction in a given year?

2. Calculate the number of farmer-days for each individual market identified in question 1 by multiplying the number of days per year the market is open by the average number of farm vendors who sell food at the market on a given day (do not include vendors who only sell crafts or packaged foods).

3. Add the total number of farmer-days for each farmers market to calculate the total annual farmer-days.

4. What is the total population within your local jurisdiction? Divide this number by 10,000.

5. Divide the total annual farmer-days (answer to item 3) by the answer to item 4.

Example:

1. Three farmers markets operated in local jurisdiction in 2008
2. Market #1: open 52 days per year x 10 farm vendors per day = 520 farmer-days
3. Market #2: open 30 days x 6 farm vendors = 180 farmer-days
4. Market #3: open 25 days x 16 farm vendors = 400 farmer-days
5. 520 + 180 + 400 = 1,100 total annual farmer-days
6. 25,000 residents / 10,000 = 2.5
7. 1,100 / 2.5 = 440 total annual farmer-days per 10,000 residents

Data Sources

- Farmers market manager(s)
- Business license official or office
- Chamber of Commerce
- County extension office: <http://www.csrees.usda.gov/qlinks/partners/state_partners.html>

STRATEGY 6: PROVIDE INCENTIVES FOR THE PRODUCTION, DISTRIBUTION, AND PROCUREMENT OF FOODS FROM LOCAL FARMS

Currently, the United States does not produce enough fruits, vegetables, whole grains, and dairy products for all U.S. citizens to eat the quantities of these foods recommended by the USDA Dietary Guidelines for Americans (Buzby, Wells, & Vocke, 2006). Increasing the production, distribution, and procurement of food from local farms might expand the capacity of the food system to produce sufficient quantities of healthier foods and to improve food security within local communities.

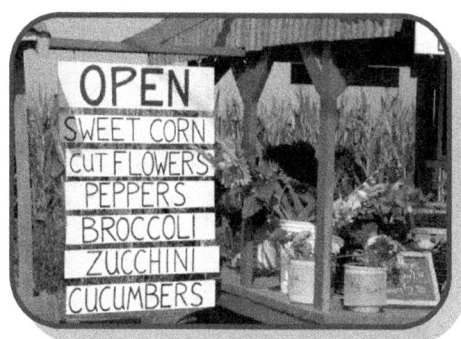

Community Examples

- The Hartford Food System (HFS) in Connecticut is a nonprofit organization working to create an equitable and sustainable food system that addresses the underlying causes of hunger and poor nutrition facing low-income and elderly residents. In addition to developing innovative projects and initiatives that tackle food cost, access, and nutrition, the organization actively participates in public policy initiatives aimed at increasing production, distribution, and procurement of foods from local farms at the local, State, and Federal Government levels (Feenstra, 1997).

- The New North Florida Cooperative (NNFC) serves as a regional lead agency for the National Farm to School Network and is the hub for farm-to-school activities in the southern region of the United States. The mission of NNFC is to facilitate the sale of locally grown produce to local school districts for school lunch and breakfast programs by acting as an intermediary between local farmers and school districts. The cooperative markets, handles, processes, and delivers fresh produce on behalf of participating local farmers at competitive prices so schools are not paying more to buy local. To date, the cooperative has served fresh fruits and vegetables to over one million students in 72 school districts (Holmes, 2009).

Resources

- Buck, M. (2007). *A guide to developing a sustainable food purchasing policy.* Portland, OR: The Food Alliance. Available online at: <www.sustainablefoodpolicy.org/SustainableFoodPolicyGuide.pdf>

- Herrera, H. (2006). *Building local food systems: A planning guide.* Rochester, NY: Center for Popular Research, Education and Policy and New York Sustainable Agriculture Working Group. Available online at: <http://www.nysawg.org/pdf/Local_Food_Planning_Guide_v2.pdf>

- Pothukuchi, K. (2007). *Building community food security: Lessons from Community Food Projects 1999–2003.* Venice, CA: Community Food Security Coalition. Available online at: <www.foodsecurity.org/BuildingCommunityFoodSecurity.pdf>

- Strategic Alliance ENACT. (n.d.). *Connect locally grown food to local food retail establishments.* Retrieved April 13, 2009, from: <http://www.preventioninstitute.org/sa/enact/neighborhood/localfood.php>

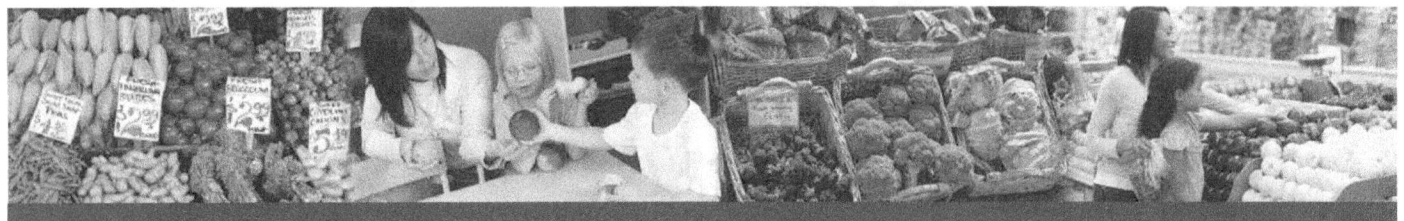

MEASURE 6:
Local government has a policy that encourages the production, distribution, or procurement of food from <u>local farms</u> in the local jurisdiction.

Data Collection Questions

1. Does your local government have a policy that encourages the production, distribution, or procurement of food from local farms?

    1a. If you answered yes to question 1, which of the following incentive(s) are offered to local farmers?

    - Purchasing electronic bank transfer (EBT) machines for farmers' markets
    - Farm-to-school programs
    - Farmland preservation
    - Marketing of local crops within the jurisdiction
    - Allowing farm stands
    - Support for grower cooperatives for smaller farms
    - Other

    1b. Is there a State policy or requirement that encourages the production, distribution, or procurement of food from local farms that applies to your local jurisdiction?

Data Sources

- Office that maintains government-wide policies (e.g., city/county manager's office, mayor's office)
- Central budget office or budget director
- County extension service: <http://www.csrees.usda.gov/qlinks/partners/state_partners.html>

Category 2: Strategies to Support Healthy Food and Beverage Choices

Strategy 7: Restrict Availability of Less Healthy Foods and Beverages in Public Service Venues

Research has shown that the availability of less healthy foods in schools is inversely associated with fruit and vegetable consumption and is positively associated with fat intake among students (Kubik, Lytle, Hannan, Perry, & Story, 2003). Schools can restrict the availability of less healthy foods by setting standards for the types of foods sold, restricting access to vending machines, banning snack foods and food as rewards in classrooms, or prohibiting food sales at certain times of the school day. Other public service venues that can restrict the availability of less healthy foods include afterschool programs, regulated child care centers, community recreational facilities (e.g., parks, swimming pools), city and county buildings, and prisons and juvenile detention centers.

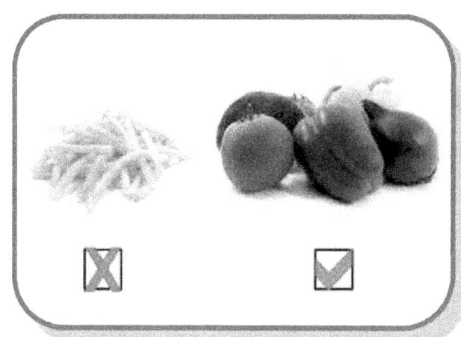

Community Examples

- The city of Baldwin Park, California, established nutrition standards for all snack foods and beverages sold in over 30 afterschool programs (including snack offerings in vending machines). The afterschool nutrition standards primarily focus on eliminating less healthy snacks and beverages that exceed recommended fat, calorie, and sugar intake for school-aged children (Healthy Eating Active Communities, 2007).

- In 2003, Arkansas passed comprehensive legislation to combat childhood obesity. One component of Act 1220 prohibits student access to food and beverage vending machines in all Arkansas elementary schools. The fourth annual evaluation of the law found a significant increase in policies to prohibit the sale of "junk foods" in schools and less availability of high-fat, high-sugar items and more availability of healthy food and beverage options in school vending machines (University of Arkansas for Medical Sciences, 2008).

- The Vista Unified School District of California implemented a vending machine policy that eliminated less healthy food options and replaced them with healthier choices at a local high school. Chips and candy were replaced with foods such as fresh fruits, vegetables, and yogurt; sodas were eliminated in favor of water, juices, and sports drinks. Vending machine sales increased significantly after policy implementation, from $9,000 to $41,000 annually (Coalition on Children and Weight San Diego, 2007).

Resources

- Center for Science in the Public Interest. (2003). *School foods tool kit*. Washington, DC: Author. Available online at: <http://www.cspinet.org/schoolfoodkit/>

- Samuels and Associates. (2006). *Competitive foods: Policy brief*. Oakland, CA: Author. Available online at: <http://www.calendow.org/uploadedFiles/competitive_foods_brief.pdf>

- U.S. Department of Agriculture. (2005). *Making it happen: School nutrition success stories*. Washington, DC: Author. Available online at: <http://www.fns.usda.gov/TN/Resources/makingithappen.html>

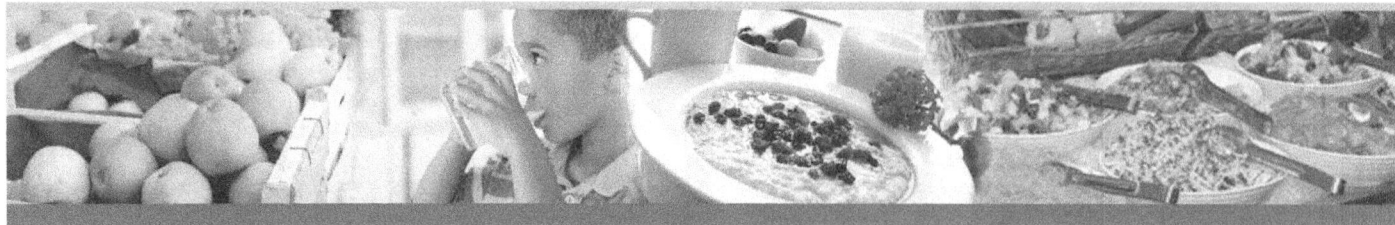

MEASURE 7: A policy exists that prohibits the sale of <u>less healthy foods and beverages</u> within <u>local government facilities</u> in a local jurisdiction or on public school campuses during the school day within the <u>largest school district in a local jurisdiction</u>.

Data Collection Questions

1. Does your local government have a policy that prohibits the sale of less healthy foods and beverages in local government facilities?

    1a. If you answered yes to question 1, to which of the following types of facilities does your local government's policy regarding the sale of less healthy foods and beverages apply?
    - Administrative office facilities
    - 24-hour "dormitory-type" facilities
    - Health care facilities
    - Recreation/community center facilities
    - Detention facilities

    1b. Is there a State policy or requirement regarding the sale of less healthy foods and beverages that applies to your local jurisdiction?

2. Does the largest school district located within the local jurisdiction have a policy that prohibits the sale of less healthy foods and beverages on public school campuses during the school day?

    2a. If you answered yes to question 2, please describe the school district's policy.

Data Sources

- Local government office that maintains government policies
- School district administrative offices

STRATEGY 8: INSTITUTE SMALLER PORTION SIZE OPTIONS IN PUBLIC SERVICE VENUES

Research has documented a relationship between food portion sizes and energy intake (Kral & Rolls, 2004; Rolls, Roe, & Meengs, 2006). Portion size is the amount (e.g., weight, calorie content, or volume) of a single food item served in a single eating occasion. Local governments can regulate food portion sizes served within public service venues such as regulated child care centers, community recreational facilities (e.g., parks, recreation centers, playgrounds, and swimming pools), city and county buildings, and prisons and juvenile detention centers.

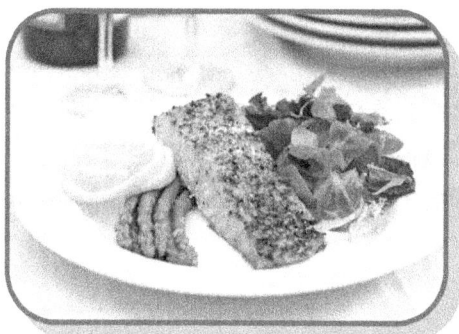

Community Examples

Although the following two examples describe programs that target private restaurants, they may serve as models for local communities that wish to promote greater access to healthy portion sizes in public service venues.

❖ The Texas Department of State Health Services developed the *Tex Plate* program to assist Texas restaurants in serving healthier portion sizes to consumers. Participating restaurants receive specialized 9-inch plates that indicate proper portions of key food groups such as vegetables, protein, and whole grains. The program is designed to encourage participating restaurants to increase the vegetable portion of the meal and decrease the entrée and starch portions of the meal (Texas Department of State Health Services, 2008).

❖ The Colorado Department of Public Health and Environment (CDPHE) implements the *Small Steps for Healthy Leaps* program to encourage restaurants to promote healthier food options for customers. One aspect of the program is the "Take ½ to Go" campaign, in which participating restaurants provide customers the option of placing half of their meal in a to-go box, while enjoying the other half at the restaurant (Live Well Colorado, n.d.).

Resources

❖ Center for Science in the Public Interest. (2003). *School foods tool kit*. Washington, DC: Author. Available online at: <http://www.cspinet.org/schoolfoodkit/>

❖ Centers for Disease Control and Prevention. (2007). *Do increased portion sizes affect how much we eat? Research to Practice Series* (No. 2). Atlanta, GA: Author. Available online at: <http://www.cdc.gov/nccdphp/dnpa/nutrition/pdf/portion_size_research.pdf>

❖ U.S. Department of Agriculture. (2005). *Making It Happen! School nutrition success stories*. Alexandria, VA: Author. Available online at: <http://www.fns.usda.gov/TN/Resources/makingithappen.html>

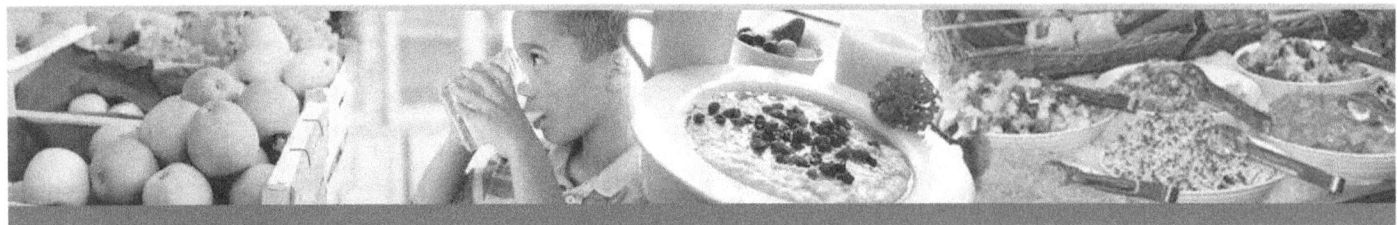

MEASURE 8:

Local government has a policy to limit the <u>portion size</u> of any entree (including sandwiches and entrée salads) by either reducing the standard portion size of entrees or offering smaller portion sizes in addition to standard portion sizes within <u>local government facilities</u> within a local jurisdiction.

Data Collection Questions

1. Does your local government have a policy to limit the portion size of any entree (including sandwiches and entrée salads) by either reducing the standard portion size of entrees or offering smaller portion sizes in addition to standard portion sizes sold within local government facilities?

    1a. If you answered yes to question 1, to which of the following types of facilities does your local government's policy regarding portion sizes apply?

    - Administrative office facilities
    - 24-hour "dormitory-type" facilities
    - Health care facilities
    - Recreation/community center facilities
    - Detention facilities
    - Other facilities

    1b. Is there a State policy or requirement regarding food portion sizes that applies to your local jurisdiction?

Data Sources

- Office that maintains government-wide policies (e.g., city/county manager's office, mayor's office)
- Facilities Management Department
- Purchasing staff person who manages the food service or vending contract for jurisdiction

STRATEGY 9: LIMIT ADVERTISEMENTS OF LESS HEALTHY FOODS AND BEVERAGES

Television advertising influences children to prefer and request high-calorie and low-nutrient foods and beverages and influences consumption among children between the ages of 2 and 11 years (IOM, 2006). Legislation to limit advertising of less healthy foods and beverages is usually introduced at the Federal or State level. However, local governing bodies, such as district-level school boards, might have the authority to limit advertisements of less healthy foods and beverages in areas within their jurisdiction (Joint Center for Political and Economic Studies and PolicyLink, 2004).

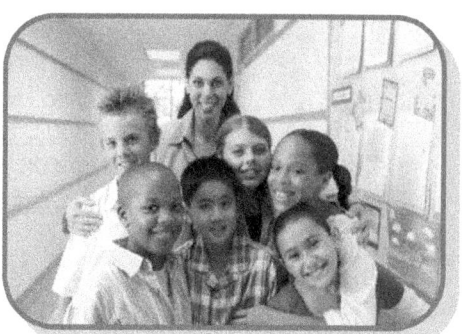

Community Examples

- In 1999, San Francisco County passed the Commercial Free Schools Act which prohibits the San Francisco Unified School District from entering into exclusive contracts with soft drink or snack food companies and restricts advertising of commercial products in the school district (Strategic Alliance ENACT, 1999).

- The Mercedes Independent School District in Mercedes, Texas, adopted a comprehensive Student Nutrition/Wellness Plan in 2005 which includes a marketing component. The policy states that schools will promote healthy food choices and will not allow advertising that promotes less nutritious food choices. The plan also defines and prohibits possession of foods of minimal nutritional value at school (Mercedes Independent School District, 2005).

Resources

- Berkeley Media Studies Group. (2006). *Fighting junk food marketing to kids: A toolkit for advocates.* Berkeley, CA: Author. Available online at: <http://www.bmsg.org/pdfs/BMSG_Junk_Food_toolkit.pdf>

- California Project LEAN. (2007). *Captive KIDS. Selling obesity at schools: An action guide to stop the marketing of unhealthy foods & beverages in school.* Sacramento, CA: Author. Available online at: <http://www.californiaprojectlean.org/Assets/1019/files/CK2007.pdf>

- National Policy & Legal Analysis Network to Prevent Childhood Obesity. (n.d.). *District policy restricting food and beverage advertising on school grounds.* Available online at: <http://www.nplanonline.org/files/DistPlcy_Food-Bev_Advrtsng_FINAL.pdf>

- Samuels, S., Craypo, L., Dorfman, L., Purciel, M., & Standish, M. (2003). *Food and beverage industry marketing practices aimed at children: Developing strategies for preventing obesity and diabetes.* San Francisco, CA: The California Endowment. Available online at: <http://epsl.asu.edu/ceru/Articles/CERU-0311-208-OWI.pdf>

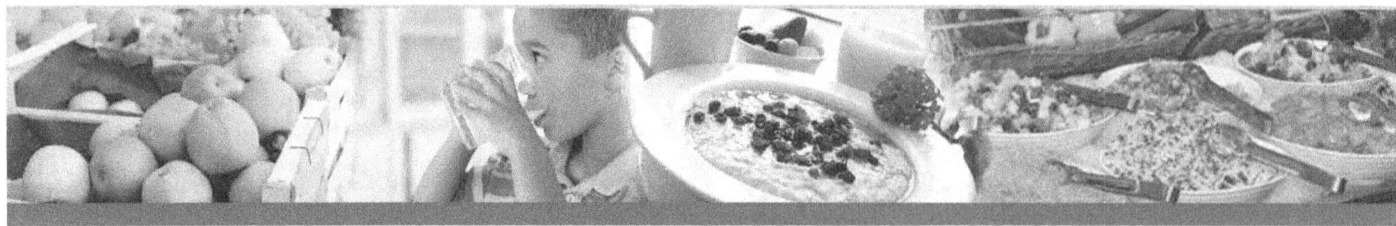

MEASURE 9:

A policy exists that limits advertising and promotion of <u>less healthy foods and beverages</u> within <u>local government facilities</u> in a local jurisdiction or on public school campuses during the school day within the <u>largest school district in a local jurisdiction</u>.

Data Collection Questions

1. Does your local government have a policy that prohibits advertising and promotion of less healthy foods and beverages within local government facilities?

   1a. If you answered yes to question 1, does your local government's policy regarding advertising and promotion of less healthy food and beverages apply to any of the following types of facilities?

   - Administrative office facilities
   - 24-hour "dormitory-type" facilities
   - Health care facilities
   - Recreation/community center facilities
   - Detention facilities
   - Other facilities

   1b. Is there a State policy or requirement that limits advertising of less healthy food and beverages that applies to your local jurisdiction?

2. Does the largest school district located within the local jurisdiction have a policy that limits advertising and promotion of less healthy food and beverages on public school campuses during the school day?

   2a. If you answered yes to question 2, please describe the school district's policy.

Data Sources

- Office that maintains government-wide policies (e.g., city/county manager's office, mayor's office)
- Facilities Management Department
- Purchasing staff person who manages the food service or vending contract for jurisdiction
- School district administrative offices

Strategy 10: Discourage Consumption of Sugar-Sweetened Beverages

Consumption of sugar-sweetened beverages (e.g., carbonated soft drinks, sports drinks, flavored/sweetened milk, and fruit drinks) among children has increased dramatically since the 1970s and is associated with higher daily caloric intake and greater risk of obesity among children and adolescents (CDC, 2006). Schools and group day care centers contribute to the problem by serving and/or allowing children to purchase sugar-sweetened beverages. Policies that restrict the availability of sugar-sweetened beverages and 100% fruit juice in schools and group day care centers may discourage the consumption of sugar-sweetened beverages among children.

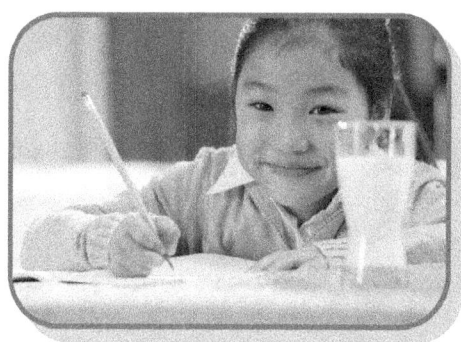

Community Examples

❖ In 2002, the Los Angeles Unified School District adopted the Motion to Promote Healthy Beverage Sales. The motion bans the sale of soft drinks on school campuses; prohibits schools from entering into new or extended sales contracts of unapproved beverages; allows only approved beverages to be sold in vending machines, cafeterias, and student stores; monitors compliance through an audit program; disseminates information on healthy beverage sale options; and develops a new revenue model to make up for anticipated net loss of Associated Student Body monies related to the ban on soft drinks (LAUSD, 2002).

❖ In 2006, the New York City Board of Health adopted regulations that provide nutrition standards and limit the serving size for beverages served to children in licensed day care centers. Specifically, the New York City Health Code prohibits serving beverages with added sweeteners and limits the serving size of 100% fruit juice to 6 ounces per day for children 8 months of age and older. When milk is served, children 2 years of age and older must receive low-fat 1% or nonfat milk and water must be made easily available to children throughout the day (New York City Department of Health and Mental Hygiene, 2006).

Resources

❖ Alliance for a Healthier Generation. (n.d.). *Alliance school beverage guidelines toolkit.* Retrieved April 13, 2009, from: <http://www.healthiergeneration.org/beveragekit>

❖ Centers for Disease Control and Prevention. (2006). *Does drinking beverages with added sugars increase the risk of overweight? Research to Practice Series* (No. 3). Atlanta, GA: Author. Available online at: <http://www.cdc.gov/nccdphp/dnpa/nutrition/pdf/r2p_sweetend_beverages.pdf>

❖ National Policy & Legal Analysis Network to Prevent Childhood Obesity. (2009). *Developing a healthy beverage vending agreement.* Available online at: <http://www.nplanonline.org/files/HealthyVendngAgrmnt_FactSheet_FINAL_090311.pdf>

❖ Strategic Alliance ENACT. (n.d.). *Eliminate exclusive beverage contracts that require the marketing of unhealthy beverages.* Retrieved April 13, 2009, from: <http://www.preventioninstitute.org/sa/enact/school/beverage_contracts_4b.php>

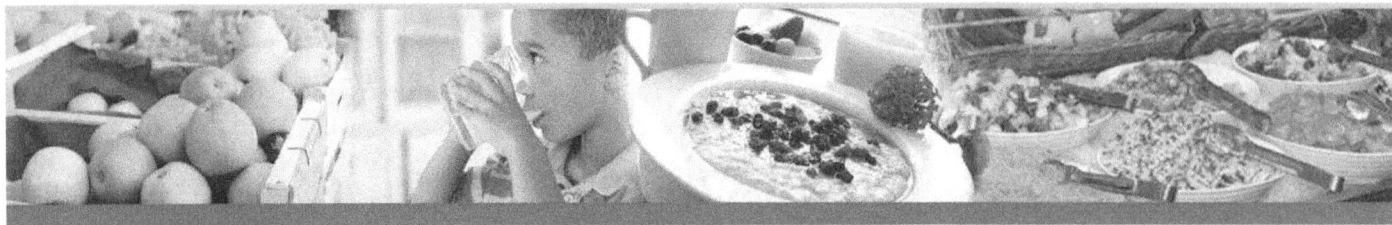

MEASURE 10:

Licensed child care facilities within the local jurisdiction are required to ban <u>sugar-sweetened beverages</u>, including flavored/sweetened milk, and limit the portion size of 100% juice.

Data Collection Questions

1. Are all licensed child care facilities in your local jurisdiction required to ban sugar-sweetened beverages, including flavored/sweetened milk?

    1a. If you answered yes to question 1, is the requirement the result of a local policy or requirement, a State policy or requirement, or some other policy or requirement?

    - Local policy or requirement
    - State policy or requirement
    - Other policy or requirement (please explain)

2. Are all licensed child care facilities in your local jurisdiction required to limit the portion size of 100% juice?

    2a. If you answered yes to question 2, is the requirement the result of a local policy or requirement, a State policy or requirement, or some other policy or requirement?

    - Local policy or requirement
    - State policy or requirement
    - Other policy or requirement (please explain)

Data Sources

- State and local child care licensing authorities

CATEGORY 3:
STRATEGY TO ENCOURAGE BREASTFEEDING

STRATEGY 11: INCREASE SUPPORT FOR BREASTFEEDING

Research has shown that breastfeeding provides a significant degree of protection against childhood obesity (IOM, 2005). Despite the advantages of breastfeeding, many women who work outside the home must bottle-feed their babies because their work setting does not provide time or private space to breastfeed or to pump breast milk. State and local governments can offer incentives to private businesses to accommodate breastfeeding among employees; they can also set policies that require government facilities to support breastfeeding among female employees.

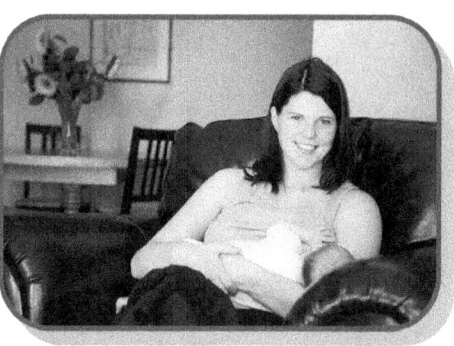

Community Examples

❖ In 1998, California passed the *Breastfeeding at Work* law, which requires all employers to ensure that employees are provided with adequate facilities for breastfeeding or expressing milk. In 2002, the State passed *Lactation Accommodation*, which expands prior workplace provisions to require adequate break time and space for breastfeeding or milk expression, with a violation penalty of $100 (Shealy, Li, Benton-Davis, & Grummer-Strawn, 2005).

❖ In 2008, Navajo Nation lawmakers passed a bill that requires employers on the reservation to provide a place for working mothers to breastfeed. The Navajo Nation Healthy Start Act allows mothers unpaid time during work hours to breastfeed their children or to use a breast pump (Fonseca, 2008).

Resources

❖ Centers for Disease Control and Prevention. (2007). *Does breastfeeding reduce the risk of pediatric overweight? Research to Practice Series* (No. 4). Atlanta, GA: Author. Available online at:
<http://www.cdc.gov/nccdphp/dnpa/nutrition/pdf/breastfeeding_r2p.pdf>

❖ Shealy, K., Li, R., Benton-Davis, S., & Grummer-Strawn, L. (2005). *The CDC guide to breastfeeding interventions*. Atlanta, GA: Centers for Disease Control and Prevention. Available online at:
<http://www.cdc.gov/breastfeeding/pdf/breastfeeding_interventions.pdf>

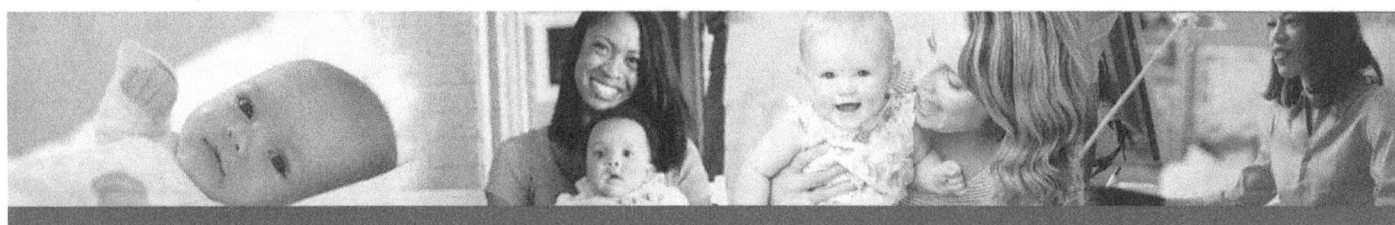

MEASURE 11:

Local government has a policy requiring <u>local government facilities</u> to provide breastfeeding accommodations for employees that include both time and designated space for breastfeeding and expressing breast milk during working hours.

Data Collection Questions

1. Does your local government have a policy requiring local government facilities to provide breastfeeding accommodations for employees, including both time and designated space for breastfeeding during working hours?

    1a. If you answered yes to question 1, to which of the following types of facilities does your local government's policy regarding breastfeeding accommodations apply?

    - Administrative office facilities
    - 24-hour "dormitory-type" facilities
    - Health care facilities
    - Recreation/community center facilities
    - Detention facilities
    - Other facilities

    1b. Is there a State policy or requirement regarding breastfeeding accommodations for government employees that applies to your local jurisdiction?

Data Sources

- Office that maintains government-wide policies (e.g., city/county manager's office, mayor's office)
- Facilities Management Department

CATEGORY 4: STRATEGIES TO ENCOURAGE PHYSICAL ACTIVITY OR LIMIT SEDENTARY ACTIVITY AMONG CHILDREN AND YOUTH

STRATEGY 12: REQUIRE PHYSICAL EDUCATION IN SCHOOLS

Evidence suggests that school-based physical education (PE) increases students' level of physical activity and improves physical fitness (Zaza, Briss, & Harris, 2005). The National Association for Sport and Physical Education (NASPE) and the American Heart Association (AHA) recommend that "all elementary school students should participate in at least 150 minutes per week of physical education, and all middle and high school students should participate in at least 225 minutes of physical education per week, for the entire school year" (NASPE & AHA, 2006, p. 2). Although school administrators express concerns that PE classes compete with traditional academic curricula, the Task Force for Community Preventive Services found no evidence that time spent in PE classes harms academic performance (Zaza et al., 2005).

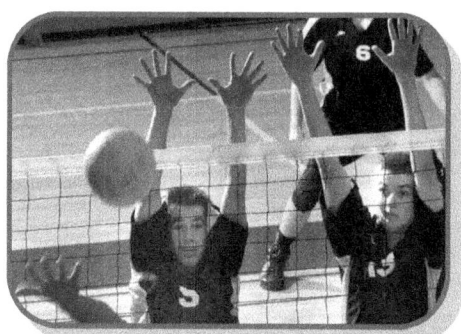

Community Examples

❖ In 2006, West Virginia enacted Senate Bill 785, which calls for the Department of Education to establish a requirement that every student enrolled in a public school participate in PE classes during the school year. The bill also specified participation times for PE classes by grade level. For example, elementary school students are required to participate in at least 30 minutes of PE class 3 days a week, middle school students are required to participate in at least one full period of PE each school day for a semester, and high school students are required to complete no less than one full course credit of PE class prior to graduation (Winterfeld, 2007).

❖ In 2007, the State of Mississippi passed the Mississippi Healthy Students Act, which includes a requirement for public schools to provide 150 minutes per week of physical activity-based instruction and 45 minutes per week of health education in grades K–8. The Act also requires 60 hours per year of physical education and 60 hours per year of health education in grades 9 thru 12 to meet graduation requirements (Mississippi Office of Healthy Schools, 2007).

Resources

❖ Partnership for Prevention. (2008). *School-based physical education: Working with schools to increase physical activity among children and adolescents in physical education classes*. Washington, DC: Author. Available online at: <http://www.prevent.org/actionguides/SchoolPE.pdf>

❖ Pennsylvania Advocates for Nutrition and Activity. (n.d.). *Physical activity action kit for change*. Retrieved April 13, 2009, from: <http://www.panaonline.org/programs/khz/actionkits/pak/intro.php>

❖ Strategic Alliance ENACT. (n.d.). *Meet or exceed requirements for minimum minutes of quality physical education*. Retrieved April 13, 2009, from: <http://www.preventioninstitute.org/sa/enact/school/physical_education.php>

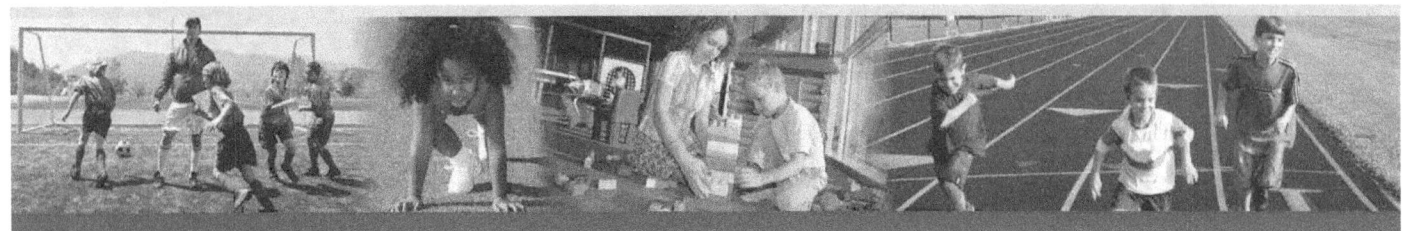

MEASURE 12:

The <u>largest school district located within the local jurisdiction</u> has a policy that requires a minimum of 150 minutes per week of physical education in public elementary schools and a minimum of 225 minutes per week of physical education in public middle schools and high schools throughout the school year.

Data Collection Questions

1. Does the largest school district located within the local jurisdiction have a policy that requires a minimum of 150 minutes per week of daily physical education in public elementary schools throughout the school year?

    1a. For each grade included in your elementary school system, is there a minimum requirement for time spent in daily physical education per week? If yes, what is the minimum weekly requirement in minutes per grade?

2. Does the largest school district located within the local jurisdiction have a policy that requires a minimum of 225 minutes per week of daily physical education in public middle and high schools throughout the school year?

    2a. For each grade included in your middle school and high school system, is there a minimum requirement for time spent in daily physical education per week? If yes, what is the minimum weekly requirement in minutes per grade?

Data Sources

- School district administrative offices: <http://nces.ed.gov/ccd/districtsearch/index.asp?start=0&ID2=1301740>
- School district's Department of Physical Education

STRATEGY 13: INCREASE THE AMOUNT OF PHYSICAL ACTIVITY IN PHYSICAL EDUCATION PROGRAMS IN SCHOOLS

Even when physical education (PE) classes are required in school, students are not necessarily physically active during those classes, particularly in the absence of high-quality curricula or well-trained PE teachers. Increasing the amount of time students spend engaged in physical activity during school-based PE classes might increase physical activity among children.

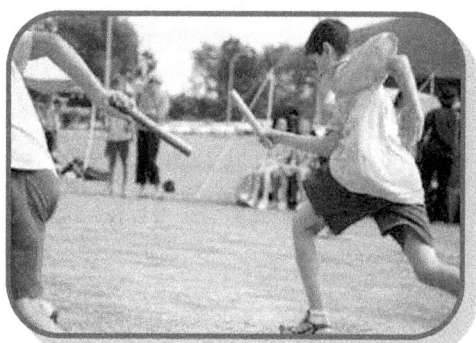

Community Examples

- Owensboro, Kentucky, overhauled its school-based PE curriculum after a study found that 60% of the Owensboro-area population was obese or overweight. A partnership was formed between the city's hospitals and schools and $750,000 was donated to equip 11 school-based fitness centers with treadmills, stationary bikes, rowing machines, and weightlifting stations. PE teachers were trained using "new PE" techniques, which stress the importance of keeping students physically active for at least 30- to 60-minute increments during class time (Weir, 2004).

- Equestrian Trails Elementary School, located in Wellington, Florida, received a STARS award from the National Association for Sport and Physical Education in recognition of its outstanding PE program. The PE staff at Equestrian Trails Elementary designed a yearly plan of instruction using physical activity and fitness components as the primary foundation for its curriculum. The curriculum teaches students the basic skills of several movement forms, including team, dual, and individual sports, and dance (National Association for Sport and Physical Education, n.d.).

Resources

- Centers for Disease Prevention and Prevention. (2006). *Physical education curriculum analysis tool.* Atlanta, GA: Author. Available online at: <http://www.cdc.gov/HealthyYouth/PECAT/pdf/PECAT.pdf>

- Partnership for Prevention. (2008). *An action guide: Working with schools to increase physical activity among children and adolescents in physical education classes.* Washington, DC: Author. Available online at: <http://www.prevent.org/actionguides/SchoolPE.pdf>

- Pennsylvania Advocates for Nutrition and Activity. (n.d.). *Physical activity action kit for change.* Retrieved April 19, 2009 from: <http://www.panaonline.org/programs/khz/actionkits/pak/intro.php>

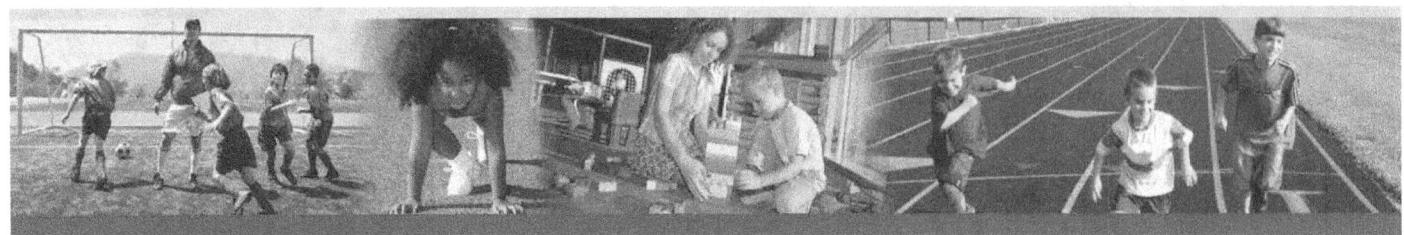

MEASURE 13:

The <u>largest school district located within the local jurisdiction</u> has a policy that requires K–12 students to be physically active for at least 50% of time spent in physical education classes in public schools.

Data Collection Questions

1. Does the largest school district located within the local jurisdiction have a policy that requires students in all grades (K–12) to be physically active for at least 50% of time spent in physical education classes in public schools?

Data Sources

- School district administrative offices: <http://nces.ed.gov/ccd/districtsearch/index.asp?start=0&ID2=1301740>
- School district's Department of Physical Education

STRATEGY 14: INCREASE OPPORTUNITIES FOR EXTRACURRICULAR PHYSICAL ACTIVITY

Children and families need places and opportunities to be physically active outside of school hours as part of a healthy lifestyle. One way to increase opportunities for physical activity is to ensure that existing recreational facilities, such as school gyms and playgrounds, are open to the public. In addition, more communities and school districts are entering joint use agreements to develop new recreational facilities that can be shared by schools and the general public.

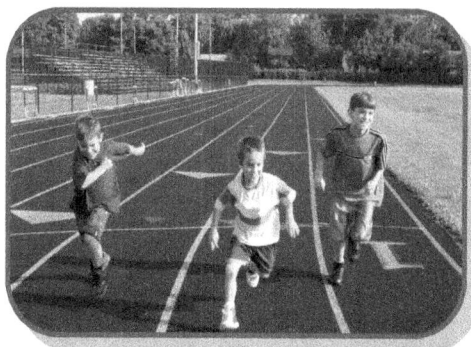

Community Examples

- The city of Eugene, Oregon, and the Bethel School District pooled their resources to purchase and develop a 70-acre parcel of land. The property now includes a 35-acre site for Meadow View School and 35 acres for Bethel Community Park, which includes wetlands, a running path, ball fields, and a skate/community park. Many students can walk through the park to get to school (Oregon Transportation and Growth Management Program, 2005).

- Pitt County, North Carolina, formed the Community Schools and Recreation Program (CSR) in 1978 to provide recreation and physical activity opportunities for all citizens. As a result of ongoing collaboration between the CSR and the Pitt County School District, all school facilities are available for free or a small service charge to community organizations, civic groups, private nonprofit agencies, commercial businesses, faith organizations, private or commercial sport leagues, and individuals (Active Living by Design, 2006).

Resources

- National Coalition for Promoting Physical Activity. (2002). *Physical activity for youth policy initiative.* Washington, DC: Author. Available online at:
<http://www.ncppa.org/Physical%20Activity%20For%20Youth%20Policy%20Initiative.pdf>

- National Policy & Legal Analysis Network to Prevent Childhood Obesity. (n.d.). *Joint use agreement 1: Opening outdoor school facilities for use during non-school hours.* Available online at:
<http://nplanonline.org/files/JU1_OutdoorAreasAgrmt_FINAL_090318.pdf>

- Statewide Afterschool Networks. (n.d.). *Afterschool as a vehicle for youth obesity prevention.* Retrieved April 13, 2009 from:
<http://www.statewideafterschoolnetworks.net/resources/wellness_and_youth_obesity_prevention.html>

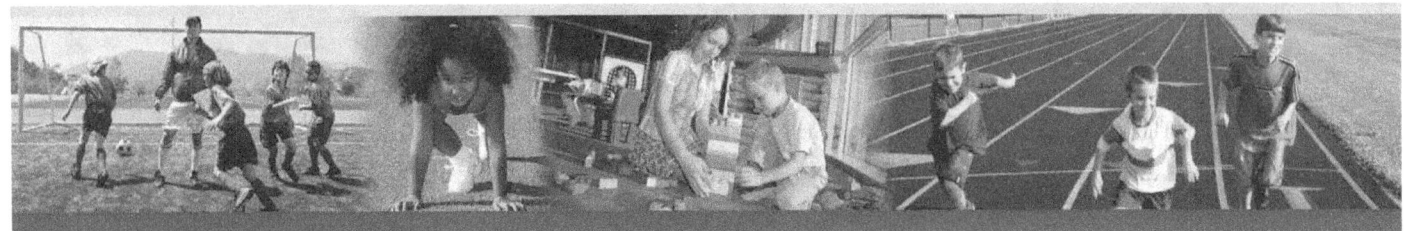

MEASURE 14:

The percentage of public schools within the <u>largest school district in a local jurisdiction</u> that allows the use of their athletic facilities by the public during nonschool hours on a regular basis.

Data Collection Questions

1. What is the total number of public elementary, middle, and high schools within the largest school district in your local jurisdiction?

2. Of the schools reported in question 1, how many schools allow the use of their athletic facilities by the public or for extracurricular physical activity programs during nonschool hours?

3. Divide the answer to question 2 by the answer to question 1 to calculate the percentage.

Data Sources

- School district administrative offices: <http://nces.ed.gov/ccd/districtsearch/index.asp?start=0&ID2=1301740>
- School district's Department of Physical Education
- Parks and Recreation Department (for list of schools that are designated parks)

STRATEGY 15: REDUCE SCREEN TIME IN PUBLIC SERVICE VENUES

When children spend too much time watching television and playing video games, they have less time for physical activity and they can be exposed to advertising of unhealthy foods and beverages (Hancox, Milne, & Poulton, 2004; Viner & Cole, 2005). The American Academy of Pediatrics recommends that children spend no more 2 hours per day watching television (American Academy of Pediatrics, 2001). State and local policymakers have an important role in limiting screen time for children in schools, day care centers, and afterschool programs.

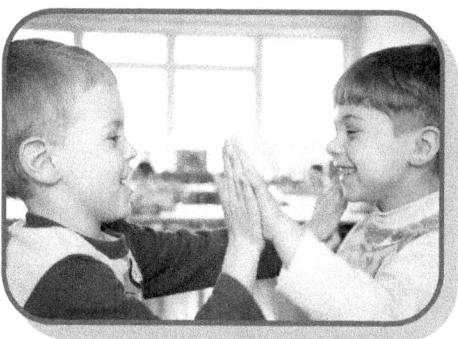

Community Examples

- In 2006, the New York City Department of Health and Mental Hygiene Board of Health implemented an amendment to the New York City Health Code, which regulates group day care in New York City. The amended article prohibits television, video, and visual recordings for children younger than 2 years of age. In addition, television, video, and visual recordings are limited to 60 minutes per day of educational programming for children 2 years or older (New York City Department of Health and Mental Hygiene, 2006).

- In 2007, Delaware's Office of Child Care Licensing promulgated regulations that set limits on the amount of screen time allowed in child care facilities. Specifically, child care facilities must limit screen time to 1 hour per day, while screen time for children younger than 2 years of age is prohibited. In addition, Delaware and Colorado are the only two States that require parental permission to use television during child care hours (Benjamin, Cradock, Walker, Slining, & Gillman, 2008).

Resources

- New York State Health Department. (2005). *NYC strategic plan for overweight and obesity prevention.* Albany, NY: Author. Available online at:
  <http://www.health.state.ny.us/prevention/obesity/strategic_plan/docs/strategic_plan.pdf>

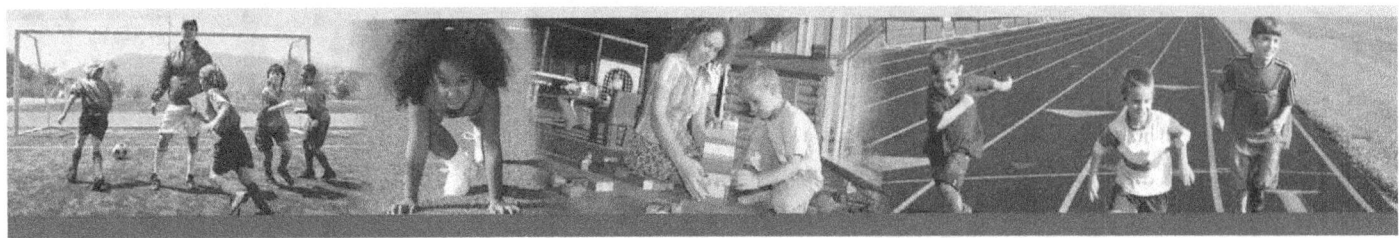

MEASURE 15:
Licensed child care facilities within the local jurisdiction are required to limit <u>screen time</u> to no more than 2 hours per day for children 2 years of age or older.

Data Collection Questions

1. Are all licensed child care venues in your local jurisdiction required to limit screen time for children 2 years of age or older to no more than 2 hours per day?

    1a. If you answered yes to question 1, is the requirement the result of a local policy or requirement, a State policy or requirement, or some other policy or requirement?
    - Local policy or requirement
    - State policy or requirement
    - Other policy or requirement (please explain)

Data Sources

- Business licensing department
- Social Services office
- Office of Child and Family Services
- Day care inspectors

CATEGORY 5: STRATEGIES TO CREATE SAFE COMMUNITIES THAT SUPPORT PHYSICAL ACTIVITY

STRATEGY 16: IMPROVE ACCESS TO OUTDOOR RECREATIONAL FACILITIES

Recreation facilities provide space for community members to engage in physical activity and include places such as parks and green space, outdoor sports fields and facilities, walking and biking trails, public pools, and community playgrounds. Access to recreation facilities is affected by proximity to homes or schools, cost, hours of operation, and transportation. Improving access to outdoor recreation facilities may increase physical activity among children and adolescents.

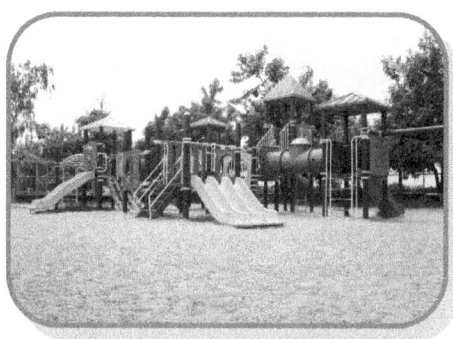

Community Examples

- The Healthy Choice Program in Duarte, California, undertook a project that rehabilitated and revitalized local hiking trails and increased access for local residents. The Fish Canyon Trail Crew, which primarily consisted of youth and adolescents, gathered to clear, widen, and repair a mile of hiking trails that led to the local park's waterfall. In addition, the program initiated the development of nine walking/jogging routes in the city and distributed maps of the routes in the community's fitness center, the Chamber of Commerce, and along the Duarte multipurpose trail. As a result of these efforts, a Teen Trekkers program was created and Bike Ride-Alongs were promoted for residents in lower-income neighborhoods (Center for Civic Partnerships, 2002).

- KaBOOM! is a national nonprofit organization that empowers local communities to build playgrounds in neighborhoods that lack play spaces for children. The KaBOOM! process helps residents of local communities bring together the capacity, resources, volunteers, and planning needed to fulfill the vision of a great place to play within walking distance of every child in America. The KaBOOM! Web site provides information and resources for community residents to apply for a KaBOOM!-led playground build or to follow detailed steps to build their own playground <http://www.kaboom.org>.

Resources

- Joint Center for Political and Economic Studies and PolicyLink. (2004). *A place for healthier living: Improving access to physical activity and healthy foods*. Washington, DC: Authors. Available online at: <http://www.policylink.org/pdfs/JointCenter-Healthyliving.pdf>

- National Coalition for Promoting Physical Activity. (2002). *Physical activity for youth policy initiative*. Washington, DC: Author. Available online at: <http://www.ncppa.org/Physical%20Activity%20For%20Youth%20Policy%20Initiative.pdf>

- Partnership for Prevention and Centers for Disease Control and Prevention. (2008). *An action guide: Facilitating development of a community trail and promoting its use to increase physical activity among youth and adults*. Available online at: <http://www.prevent.org/actionguides/CommunityTrail.pdf>

MEASURE 16: The percentage of residential parcels within a local jurisdiction that are located within a ½-mile network distance of at least one outdoor public recreational facility.

Data Collection Questions

1. What is the total number of residences within your jurisdiction?

2. Of the residences reported in question 1, how many are located within a ½-mile network distance of an outdoor public recreational facility entrance?

3. Divide the answer to question 2 by the answer to question 1 to calculate the percentage.

Data Sources

- GIS office/coordinator
- Parks and Recreation Department

Necessary GIS Functions or Layers

- GIS layer showing outdoor public recreational facilities
- GIS layer showing street networks
- GIS layer showing all parcels within the jurisdiction, with zoning classification
- Ability to calculate point to point, or point to area, network distances
- (Optional) Ability to draw buffer lines and to calculate the number of parcels that fall within the buffer

Strategy 17: Enhance Infrastructure Supporting Bicycling

Research shows a strong and significant association between bicycling infrastructure and frequency of bicycling for both recreational and commuting purposes (Dill & Carr, 2003; Staunton et al., 2003). Infrastructure that supports bicycling includes bike lanes, shared-use paths, bike routes on existing and new roads, and bike racks in the vicinity of commercial and other public spaces. Local governments have a vital role to play in developing and maintaining bicycling infrastructure for local residents.

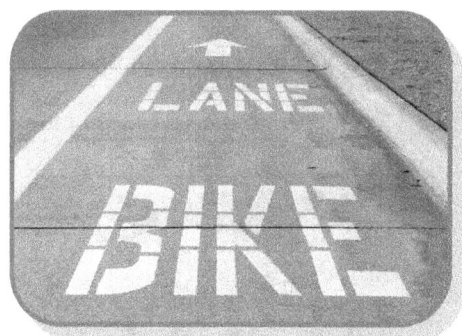

Community Examples

- In May 2005, Boulder, Colorado, was awarded Gold status as a Bicycle-Friendly Community by the League of American Bicyclists. The city committed 15% of its annual transportation budget, $3.1 million, toward bicycle enhancement and maintenance activities. More than 95% of Boulder's arterial streets have bicycle facilities and all local and regional buses are equipped with bike racks. In addition, Boulder has created an online bike routing system that provides cyclists a direct and safe bike route to travel within city limits (League of American Bicyclists, 2005).

- The National Center for Safe Routes to School provides guidance and resources to hundreds of local communities throughout the Nation to promote walking and biking to school. Marin County, California, enlisted a traffic engineer to help schools identify and create safe bike routes between residential areas and participating schools. In the first 2 years of the program, the number of children walking to school increased 64%, biking increased 114%, and carpooling increased 91% (Staunton, Hubsmith, & Kallins, 2003).

Resources

- Crump, C., & Emery, J. (2003). *The WABSA Project: Assessing and improving your community's walkability & bikeability.* University of North Carolina at Chapel Hill, School of Public Health. Available online at: <http://www.unc.edu/~jemery/WABSA/documents/wabsa%20guidebook%202003-1029.pdf>

- National Center for Bicycling and Walking. (2002). *Increasing physical activity through community design: A guide for public health practitioners.* Washington, DC: Author. Available online at: <http://www.bikewalk.org/pdfs/IPA_full.pdf>

- Pedestrian and Bicycle Information Center. (2007). *The Safe Routes to School guide.* Chapel Hill, NC: Author. Available online at: <http://www.saferoutesinfo.org/guide/pdf/SRTS-Guide_full.pdf>

- Thunderhead Alliance for Biking and Walking. (2006). *Model policy: Guide to complete streets campaigns.* Available online at: <www.thunderheadalliance.org/pdf/Guide%20Excerpts.pdf>

MEASURE 17: Total miles of designated <u>shared-use paths</u> and <u>bike lanes</u> relative to the total street miles (excluding limited access highways) that are maintained by a local jurisdiction.

Data Collection Questions

1. What is the total mileage of paved streets managed and paid for by your jurisdiction (excluding limited access highways)?

2. What is the total mileage of designated shared-use paths and bike lanes within your jurisdiction?

3. Divide the answer to question 2 by the answer to question 1 to calculate the percentage.

Data Sources

- GIS office/coordinator
- Parks and Recreation Department

Necessary GIS Functions or Layers

- Ability to calculate total street miles (less limited access highways) that are maintained by the jurisdiction
- Ability to calculate total miles of paved sidewalks, shared-use paths, and bike lanes

STRATEGY 18: ENHANCE INFRASTRUCTURE SUPPORTING WALKING

Walking is a basic form of transportation and can be an important source of daily physical activity. However, walking can be difficult for residents when communities lack sidewalks, footpaths, walking trails, and safe pedestrian street crossings. Local governments play a key role in shaping community infrastructure to support walking by promoting transit, community planning, and zoning provisions, and by retrofitting existing areas to better serve pedestrians.

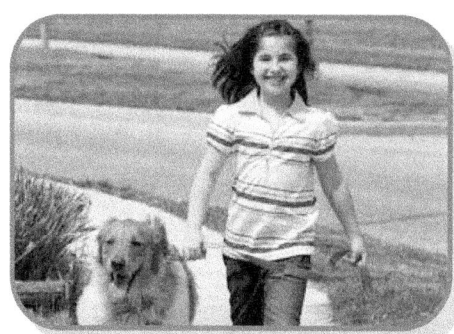

Community Examples

❖ In 2002, the City of Oakland, California, adopted a Pedestrian Master Plan which designates a network of pedestrian facilities and distinguishes segments and intersections in need of particular attention for safety enhancements. The city estimated pedestrian volumes throughout the city based on land use, population, and other network characteristics, and used these estimates in conjunction with crash data, traffic data, and community input to identify and prioritize areas with both safety problems and high pedestrian demand (City of Oakland, n.d.).

❖ In an effort to increase physical activity for residents, four towns in northern Maine created walking and biking trails from preexisting winter ski trails. The towns of Van Buren, Caribou, Stockholm, and New Sweden all had limited sidewalks or paved shoulders for community members to use. The ski trails consisted of rough brush and mud in spring, summer, and fall but are now refurbished with packed dirt and can be enjoyed by residents year-round (Healthy Maine Partnerships, 2003).

Resources

❖ Bicycle Federation of America Campaign to Make America Walkable. (1998). *Creating walkable communities: A guide for local governments*. Washington, DC: Author. Available online at: <http://www.bikewalk.org/pdfs/ncbwpubwalkablecomm.pdf>

❖ Crump, C., & Emery, J. (2003). *The WABSA project: Assessing and improving your community's walkability & bikeability*. University of North Carolina at Chapel Hill, School of Public Health. Available online at: <http://www.unc.edu/~jemery/WABSA/documents/wabsa%20guidebook%2003-1029.pdf>

❖ National Center for Bicycling and Walking. (2002). *Increasing physical activity through community design: A guide for public health practitioners*. Washington, DC: Author. Available online at: <http://www.bikewalk.org/pdfs/IPA_full.pdf>

❖ Thunderhead Alliance for Biking and Walking. (2006). *Model policy: Guide to complete streets campaigns*. Available online at: <www.thunderheadalliance.org/pdf/Guide%20Excerpts.pdf>

MEASURE 18: Total miles of paved sidewalks relative to the total street miles (excluding limited access highways) that are maintained by a local jurisdiction.

Data Collection Questions

1. What is the total mileage of paved streets managed and paid for by your jurisdiction (excluding limited access highways)?

2. What is the total mileage of paved sidewalks?

3. Divide the answer to question 2 by the answer to question 1 to calculate the percentage.

Data Sources

- GIS office/coordinator

Necessary GIS Functions or Layers

- Ability to calculate total street miles (less limited access highways) that are maintained by the jurisdiction
- Ability to calculate total miles of paved sidewalks and shared-use paths

STRATEGY 19: SUPPORT LOCATING SCHOOLS WITHIN EASY WALKING DISTANCE OF RESIDENTIAL AREAS

Walking to and from school can be a source of physical activity for children. However, fewer children are able to walk to school today because many new schools are not accessible to pedestrians due to current land use trends and policies (Environmental Protection Agency, 2003). Local governments can support locating schools within easy walking distance of residential areas by changing land use policies and/or renovating existing schools located in residential neighborhoods.

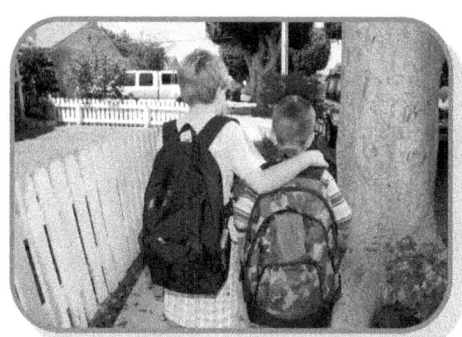

Community Examples

- In 2005, the City of Milwaukee began its Neighborhood Schools initiative. As a result of this initiative, the city decided to build six new schools from the ground up and spent millions of dollars revamping and expanding dilapidated schools that were located in and around community neighborhoods. The goals of the initiative were to reduce the number of students being bused to schools around the city and to increase the number of students walking or biking to schools that were centrally located and close to their neighborhoods (National Center for Safe Routes to School, 2007).

- The Bend-LaPine School District, in Bend City, Oregon, conducted a Sites and Facilities Study in 2000 to guide its school development master plan for the next 15 years. The study recommended building smaller school facilities, serving a maximum of 300 students, in areas more accessible to students wishing to walk or bike to school. The district opened Ensworth Elementary in 2004; of the 300 students that attend the school, 250 can walk or bike to school and only one bus is used to transport children across a busy road (Oregon Transportation and Growth Management Program, 2005).

Resources

- CDC. (n.d.). *Kids Walk-to-School: A program of the Division of Nutrition Physical Activity and Obesity.* Available online at: <http://www.cdc.gov/nccdphp/Dnpa/kidswalk>

- International City/County Management Association. (2008). *Local governments and schools: A community-oriented approach.* ICMA IQ Report 40 (Special Edition). Washington, DC: Author. Available online at: <http://www.icma.org>

- Michigan Department of Community Health. (n.d.). *Healthy communities toolkit: How you can work toward creating healthy communities.* Available online at: <http://www.mihealthtools.org/documents/HealthyCommunitiesToolkit_web.pdf>

- Oregon Transportation and Growth Management Program. (2005). *Planning for schools and liveable communities: The Oregon school siting handbook.* Salem, OR: Author. Available online at: <www.oregon.gov/LCD/TGM/docs/schoolsitinghandbook.pdf>

- PolicyLink. (2007). *The impact of the built environment on community health: The state of current practice and next steps for a growing movement.* Oakland, CA: Author. Available online at: <http://www.calendow.org/uploadedFiles/The_Built_Environment_report.pdf>

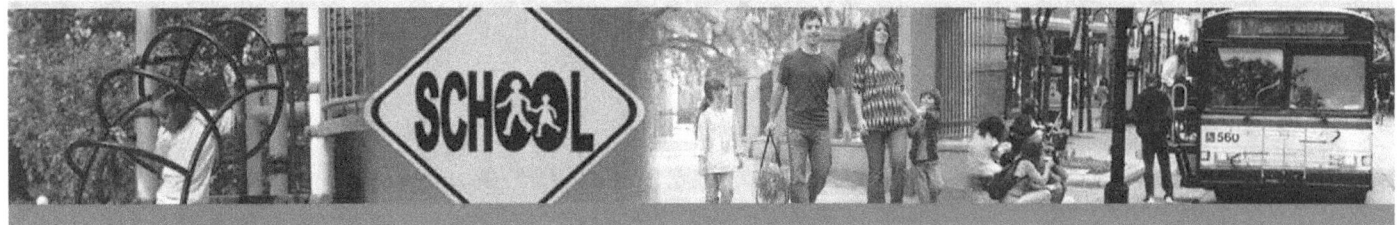

MEASURE 19:

The <u>largest school district in the local jurisdiction</u> has a policy that supports locating new schools and/or repairing or expanding existing schools, within easy walking or biking distance of residential areas.

Data Collection Questions

1. Does the largest school district in the local jurisdiction have a policy that supports locating new schools, and/or repairing or expanding existing schools, within easy walking or biking distance of residential areas?

Data Sources

- School district administrative office: <http://nces.ed.gov/ccd/districtsearch/index.asp?start=0&ID2=1301740>
- School district transportation coordinator

STRATEGY 20: IMPROVE ACCESS TO PUBLIC TRANSPORTATION

Walking to and from public transportation can help individuals attain recommended levels of daily physical activity (Besser & Dannenberg, 2005). Public transportation includes mass transit systems such as buses, light rail, street cars, commuter trains, and subways, and the infrastructure supporting these systems (e.g., transit stops and dedicated bus lanes). Improving access to public transportation may help promote more active lifestyles.

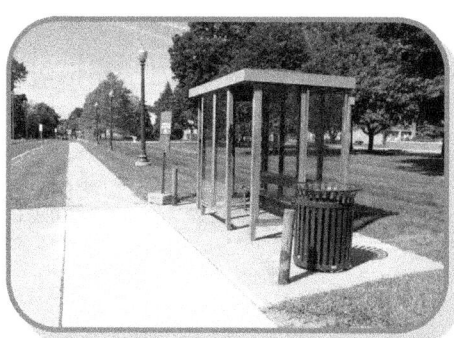

Community Examples

- Local business owners and residents of the South Park neighborhood of Tucson, Arizona, received funding from the local government and the Federal Transit Administration (FTA) to implement a series of improvements to the existing public transit system. Funds were used to install six new artistic bus shelters, new traffic signals, and additional sidewalk and curb access ramps for public transit users, bicyclers, and pedestrians. As a result of the efforts to revitalize its public transit infrastructure, South Park has experienced renewed pride in its community and helped to rebuild its local economy (Public Transportation Partnership for Tomorrow, 2008).

- The Amtrak station in Emeryville, California, is an example of transit-oriented development (TOD) which focuses on creating compact growth around transit stops as a way to increase access to public transportation. EmoryStation incorporates a 550,000-square-foot mixed-use complex surrounding a regional commuter rail line station. The station complex includes 150 units of owner-occupied lofts and townhomes, a senior living housing project, office and commercial space, and plentiful above- and below-ground parking to accommodate commuters and residents (Parker & Arrington, 2002).

Resources

- American Public Transportation Association. (n.d.). *The benefits of public transportation: The route to better personal health.* Washington, DC: Author. Available online at:
  <http://www.publictransportation.org/pdf/reports/better_health.pdf>

- McCann, B. (2006). *Community design for healthy eating: How land use and transportation solutions can help.* Princeton, NJ: Robert Wood Johnson Foundation. Available online at:
  <www.rwjf.org/files/publications/other/communitydesignhealthyeating.pdf>

- National Center for Bicycling and Walking. (2002). *Increasing physical activity through community design: A guide for public health practitioners.* Washington, DC: Author. Available online at:
  <http://www.bikewalk.org/pdfs/IPA_full.pdf>

- U.S. Department of Transportation, Federal Highway Administration. (n.d.). *Tool kit for integrating land use and transportation decision-making.* Available online at:
  <http://www.fhwa.dot.gov/planning/landuse/index.htm>

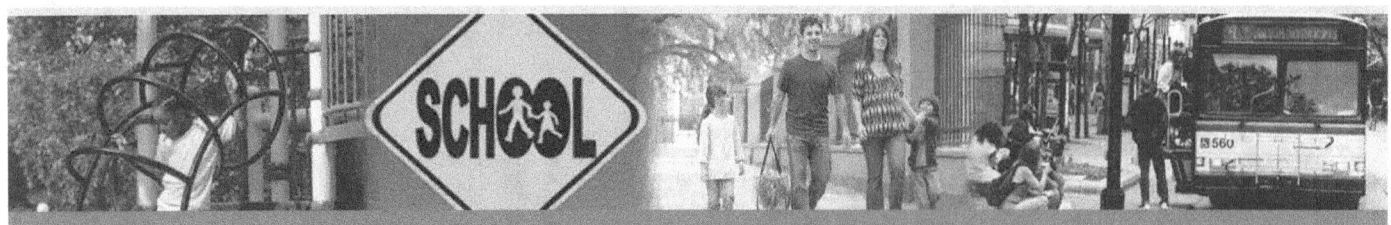

MEASURE 20:

The percentage of residential and commercial parcels in a local jurisdiction that are either located within a ¼-mile <u>network distance</u> of at least one bus stop or within a ½-mile network distance of at least one train stop (including commuter and passenger trains, light rail, subways, and street cars).

Data Collection Questions

1. How many residential parcels are in your jurisdiction?

2. How many commercial parcels are in your jurisdiction?

3. Add the answer to question 1 and the answer to question 2 to calculate the combined total of residential and commercial parcels.

4. Of the total number of combined residential and commercial parcels in your jurisdiction, how many are located either within ¼-mile network distance of a bus stop or within ½-mile network distance of a train stop?

5. Divide the answer to question 4 by the answer to item 3 to calculate the percentage.

Data Sources

- GIS office/coordinator
- Transit Service head or staff
- Liaison to the regional transit authority
- Federal Transit Administration:
  http://www.ntdprogram.gov/ntdprogram/pubs/ARM/2008/pdf/2008_Service_Module.pdf

Necessary GIS Functions or Layers

- GIS layer showing all parcels within the jurisdiction, with zoning classification
- GIS layer showing all transit stops, including buses, commuter and passenger trains, light rail, subways, and street cars
- GIS layer showing the street network
- Ability to calculate point to point, or point to area, network distances

STRATEGY 21: ZONE FOR MIXED-USE DEVELOPMENT

Mixed-use development is the combination of residential, commercial, industrial, and public land use within close proximity of one another and is associated with the number of trips people make on foot or by bicycle (Saelens, Sallis, & Frank, 2003). Zoning laws restricting the mixing of residential and nonresidential uses can be a barrier to physical activity, whereas zoning regulations that accommodate mixed land use could increase physical activity by encouraging walking and bicycling for commuting purposes.

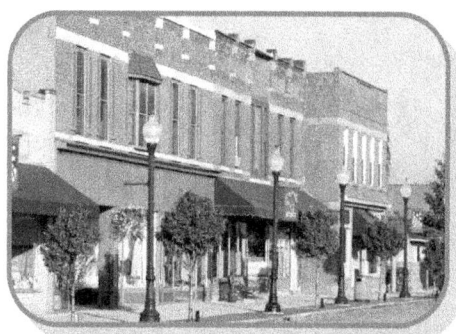

Community Examples

❖ King County, Washington, developed a comprehensive land use plan that encourages zoning for mixed-use development as a way to support active living among residents. The land use plan outlines specific design components for mixed-use developments, such as integrating retail establishments and business offices into the same buildings as residential units, ensuring the availability of parking lots or parking garages either within or close to buildings, and having safe pedestrian connections and bicycle facilities throughout the area (Metropolitan King County Council, 2006).

❖ The concept of mixed-use development is the official growth management policy for Eugene, Oregon, which focuses on integrating mixed-use developments within the city's urban growth boundary. The city's regional transportation master plan targets dozens of potential "mixed-use centers" for development into quality neighborhoods that enjoy higher densities, more transportation options, and convenient access to shopping, consumer services, and basic amenities. By combining mixed-use centers with improved transit options, the plan aims to reduce dependence on automobile travel, encourage walking, and reduce the need for costly street improvements (City of Eugene, n.d.).

Resources

❖ McCann, B. (2006). *Community design for healthy eating: How land use and transportation solutions can help.* Princeton, NJ: Robert Wood Johnson Foundation. Available online at:
<http://www.rwjf.org/files/publications/other/communitydesignhealthyeating.pdf>

❖ Michigan Department of Community Health. (n.d.). *Healthy communities toolkit: How you can work toward creating healthy communities.* Available online at:
<http://www.mihealthtools.org/documents/HealthyCommunitiesToolkit_web.pdf>

❖ National Center for Bicycling and Walking. (2002). *Increasing physical activity through community design: A guide for public health practitioners.* Washington, DC: Author. Available online at:
<http://www.bikewalk.org/pdfs/IPA_full.pdf>

❖ PolicyLink. (2007). *The impact of the built environment on community health: The state of current practice and next steps for a growing movement.* Oakland, CA: Author. Available online at:
<http://www.calendow.org/uploadedFiles/The_Built_Environment_report.pdf>

MEASURE 21:
Percentage of zoned land area (in acres) within a local jurisdiction that is zoned for <u>mixed use</u> that specifically combines residential land use with one or more commercial, institutional, or other public land uses.

Data Collection Questions

1. What is the total number of acres of zoned land within your jurisdiction?

2. Of the area reported in question 1, how many acres are zoned for mixed use (combination of residential and nonresidential)?

3. Divide the answer to question 2 by the answer to question 1.

Data Sources

- GIS office/coordinator
- Zoning administrator
- Planning department
- Land use plan administrator

Necessary GIS Functions or Layers

- GIS layer showing all parcels within the jurisdiction, with zoning classification
- Ability to calculate area in acres based on zoning classifications

STRATEGY 22: ENHANCE PERSONAL SAFETY IN AREAS WHERE PEOPLE ARE OR COULD BE PHYSICALLY ACTIVE

People may be less inclined to walk and play outdoors in neighborhoods that are perceived to be unsafe due to crime and violence (Ferreira et al., 2007). Safety considerations have been shown to affect parents' decisions to allow their children to play and walk outside (IOM, 2005). Local governments can implement efforts to improve neighborhood safety such as increasing police presence, reducing the number of abandoned buildings, and improving street lighting.

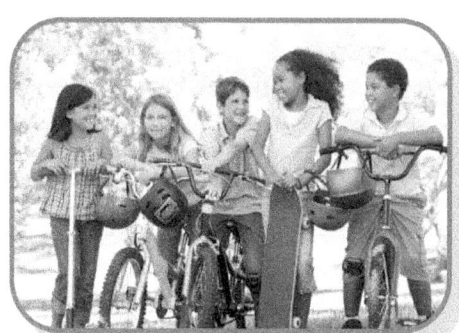

Community Examples

- In 1998, the City of Escondido, California, passed a land use policy that allows public use of private vacant lots for community purposes such as community gardens, recreational spaces, temporary public art installations, and youth recreation. The purpose of the policy is to eliminate blight and encourage walkability and physical activity among community residents by increasing their sense of personal safety in their neighborhoods (Strategic Alliance ENACT, 1998).

- Detroit, Michigan, has one of the highest home foreclosure rates in the country, resulting in a dramatic increase in the number of abandoned buildings and boarded-up homes which attract vandals and petty crime. In response, Urban Farming, an international nonprofit organization, joined forces with the local county government to transform 20 abandoned properties into active fruit and vegetable garden plots that feed the homeless and improve the aesthetic appeal of city neighborhoods. Since establishing the gardens, residents report less vandalism and blight in their community and the local county government donates water to maintain the city gardens on an ongoing basis (Bear, 2008).

Resources

- Local Initiatives Support Corporation. (2007). *Leveraging code enforcement for neighborhood safety: Insights for community developers.* New York: Author. Available online at: <http://www.lisc.org/content/publications/detail/5648>

- Prevention Institute. (2008). *Overview of the UNITY RoadMap: A framework for effective and sustainable efforts.* Available online at: <http://www.preventioninstitute.org/RoadMap.html>

MEASURE 22: Number of vacant or abandoned buildings (residential and commercial) relative to the total number of buildings located within a local jurisdiction.

Data Collection Questions

1. What is the total number of residential and commercial buildings located within your local jurisdiction?
2. Of the buildings reported in question 1, how many are vacant or abandoned?
3. Divide the answer to question 2 by the answer to question 1 to calculate the percentage.

Data Sources

- HUD & U.S. Postal Service Address Counts & Vacancies: <http://www.huduser.org/datasets/usps.html>
- GIS office/coordinator
- Zoning administrator
- Planning department

Necessary GIS Functions or Layers

- GIS layer showing individual structure information (residential structures and commercial structures)
- GIS layer showing occupancy status of structures in the jurisdiction

STRATEGY 23: ENHANCE TRAFFIC SAFETY IN AREAS WHERE PEOPLE ARE OR COULD BE PHYSICALLY ACTIVE

Traffic safety is the security of pedestrians and bicyclists from motorized traffic. Traffic safety can be enhanced by engineering streets for lower speeds or by retrofitting existing streets with traffic calming measures or improved street crossings for pedestrians. Enhancing traffic safety has been shown to be effective in increasing levels of physical activity in adults and children (Heath et al., 2006).

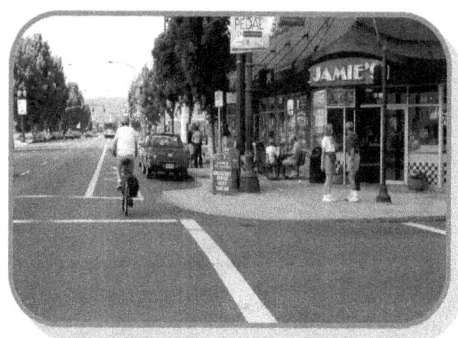

Community Examples

❖ After noting an increase in motor vehicle crashes resulting in pedestrian injuries and fatalities, a public official in Montgomery County, Maryland, appointed a 40-member Blue Ribbon Panel on Pedestrian and Traffic Safety. The panel developed an action-oriented set of recommendations to reduce pedestrian deaths and injuries and their associated economic costs by addressing ways to create pedestrian-friendly, walkable communities. The panel also developed a pedestrian safety toolbox for community planners (Montgomery County Blue Ribbon Panel on Pedestrian and Traffic Safety, 2002).

❖ In the mid-1990s, the City of West Palm Beach, Florida, adopted a downtown-wide traffic calming policy to improve street safety for nonmotorized users. The city's main streets were retrofitted with important pedestrian safety measures, including raised intersections, two-way streets, road narrowings and roundabouts to slow traffic, wide sidewalks, tree-lined streets, and shortened pedestrian crossings. As a result of these efforts, city streets are perceived as safe by pedestrians, property values more than doubled in the downtown area, and commercial retail space is 80% occupied (Lockwood & Stillings, 1998).

Resources

❖ Local Initiatives Support Corporation. (2007). *Leveraging code enforcement for neighborhood safety: Insights for community developers.* New York: Author. Available online at:
<http://www.lisc.org/content/publications/detail/5648>

❖ Montgomery County Blue Ribbon Panel on Pedestrian and Traffic Safety. (2002). *Setting safety in motion: Recommendations for creating walkable communities in Montgomery County.* Available online at:
<http://www.montgomerycountymd.gov/content/dot/dir/pedsafety/pdf/blue_ribbon_panel_final_report.pdf>

❖ Public Health Law and Policy. (n.d.). *Complete streets: Talking points.* Oakland, CA: Author. Available online at: <http://www.healthyplanning.org/factsheets/PHLP_CompleteSts.pdf>

MEASURE 23: Local government has a policy for designing and operating streets with safe access for all users that includes at least one element suggested by the National Complete Streets Coalition <www.completestreets.org>.

Data Collection Questions

1. Does your jurisdiction have a policy for designing and operating streets with safe access for all users that includes at least one of the following elements?

    - Specifies that "all users" includes pedestrians, bicyclists, transit vehicles and users, and motorists, of all ages and abilities
    - Aims to create a comprehensive, integrated, connected network
    - Recognizes the need for flexibility: that all streets are different and user needs will be balanced.
    - Is adoptable by all agencies to cover all roads
    - Applies to both new and retrofit projects, including design, planning, maintenance, and operations, for the entire right of way
    - Makes any exceptions specific and sets a clear procedure that requires high-level approval of exceptions
    - Directs the use of the latest and best design standards
    - Directs that complete streets solutions fit into the context of the community
    - Establishes performance standards with measurable outcomes

    1a. If you answered yes to question 1, which of the elements listed above does your policy include?

Data Sources

- Transportation planning office
- City/county manager's office
- City/county planning office

CATEGORY 6: STRATEGY TO ENCOURAGE COMMUNITIES TO ORGANIZE FOR CHANGE

STRATEGY 24: LOCAL GOVERNMENTS PARTICIPATE IN COMMUNITY COALITIONS OR PARTNERSHIPS TO ADDRESS OBESITY

Community coalitions consist of public- and private-sector organizations working together with individual citizens to achieve a shared goal through the coordinated use of resources, leadership, and action (IOM, 2005). The effectiveness of community coalitions stems from the multiple perspectives, talents, and expertise that are brought together to work toward a common goal. Local governments have critical perspectives and resources to share with community coalitions aiming to prevent obesity by improving the local food and physical activity environment.

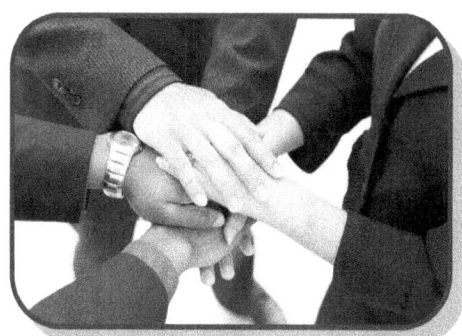

Community Examples

❖ In California, the Sonoma County Family Activity and Nutrition Task Force engages individual citizens, professionals, and community-based organizations to focus on the health, nutrition, and physical activity levels of children in the county. The Task Force promotes the availability of fruits and vegetables in local schools and public awareness of obesity-related issues and solutions (IOM, 2005).

❖ A Food Policy Council (FPC) is a type of coalition that brings together stakeholders from diverse food-related areas to examine how the food system is working. In Knoxville, Tennessee, an FPC monitors and evaluates the performance of the city's food system and recommends actions to improve it. A major accomplishment of the FPC was improving access to competitively priced nutritious foods by changing the city bus routes so that poorer inner city residents could reach outlying supermarkets (Dahlberg, 1992).

❖ PedNet Coalition in Columbia, Missouri, is a community coalition that includes 5,000 individuals and 75 businesses, government agencies, and nonprofit organizations. The goal of the coalition is to develop and restore a network of nature trails and urban "pedways" connecting residential subdivisions, worksites, shopping districts, parks, schools, and recreation centers (PedNet Coalition, 2008).

Resources

❖ Butterfoss, F., Goodman, R., & Wandersman, A. (1993). Community coalitions for prevention and health promotion. *Health Education Research: Theory and Practice, 8*(3), 315–330. Available online at: <http://her.oxfordjournals.org/cgi/reprint/8/3/315>

❖ National Coalition for Promoting Physical Activity. (n.d.). *State coalition handbook: Strategies & techniques.* Washington, DC: Author. Available online at: <http://www.ncppa.org/State%20Coalition%20Handbook%20Final.pdf>

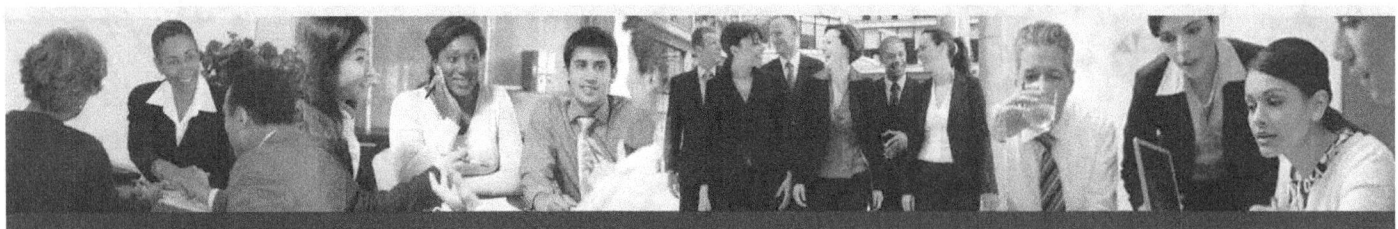

Measure 24:

Local government is an active member of at least one <u>coalition</u> or <u>partnership</u> that aims to promote environmental and policy change for active living and/or healthy eating (excluding personal health programs such as health fairs).

Data Collection Questions

1. Does your local government participate in at least one coalition or partnership that addresses active living and/or healthy eating?

    1a. If you answered yes to question 1, in how many coalitions or partnerships does your local government participate?

Data Sources

- Health department
- City/county manager's office
- Mayor's office

REFERENCES

REFERENCES

Active Living by Design. (2006). *Partnership between local school district and county open school physical activity facilities to public.* Chapel Hill, NC: Author.

American Academy of Pediatrics. (2001). Children, adolescents, and television. *Pediatrics, 107*(2), 423-426.

Anupama, J., Kalb, M., & Beery, M. (2006). *Going local: Paths to success for farm to school programs.* Los Angeles, CA: National Farm to School Program, Center for Food & Justice and Community Food Security Coalition.

Bear, C. (2008). Farms take root in Detroit's foreclosures. On *NPR Morning Edition*.

Bell, J., & Rubin, V. (2007). *Why place matters: Building a movement for healthy communities.* Oakland, CA: PolicyLink.

Benjamin, S. E., Cradock, A., Walker, E. M., Slining, M., & Gillman, M. W. (2008). Obesity prevention in child care: A review of U.S. state regulations. *BMC Public Health, 8*, 188.

Besser, L. M., & Dannenberg, A. L. (2005). Walking to public transit: Steps to help meet physical activity recommendations. *Am J Prev Med, 29*(4), 273-280.

Burton, H., & Duane, P. (2004). *Stimulating supermarket development: A new day for Philadelphia.* Philadelphia, PA: The Food Trust.

Buzby, J. C., Wells, H. F., & Vocke, G. (2006). *Possible implications for U.S. agriculture from adoption of select dietary guidelines.* Washington, DC: U.S. Department of Agriculture.

CDC. (2006). *Does drinking beverages with added sugars increase the risk of overweight? Research to Practice Series* (No. 3). Atlanta, GA: National Center for Chronic Disease Prevention and Health Promotion, Division of Nutrition and Physical Activity.

Center for Civic Partnerships. (2002). *Fresh ideas for community nutrition and physical activity.* Sacramento, CA: Public Health Institute.

City of Eugene. (n.d.). Mixed-use development in Eugene. Retrieved June 9, 2009 from http://www.eugene-or.gov/portal/server.pt?space=CommunityPage&control=SetCommunity&CommunityID=334&PageID=0

City of New York. (2009). Food retail expansion to support health. Retrieved May 18, 2009, from http://www.nyc.gov/html/misc/html/2009/fresh.shtml

City of Oakland. (n.d.). *Oakland pedestrian master plan and space syntax model.* Oakland, CA: Author.

Coalition on Children and Weight San Diego. (2007). *A call to action: Childhood obesity action plan for San Diego County.* San Diego, CA: Our Community Our Kids.

Dahlberg, K. A. (1992). *Report and recommendations on the Knoxville, Tennessee, food system.* Kalamazoo, MI: Western Michigan University, Department of Political Science.

Department of Housing and Urban Development. (1995). 24 Code of Federal Regulation, Part 81: The Secretary of HUD's Regulation of the Federal National Mortgage Association and the Federal Home Loan Mortgage Corporation (Vol. 60, pp. 61854-61855): Federal Register.

Dill, J., & Carr, T. (2003). Bicycle commuting and facilities in major U.S. cities: If you build them, commuters will use them. *Transportation Research Record, 1829*, 116-123.

Drewnowski, A. (2004). Obesity and the food environment: Dietary energy density and diet costs. *Am J Prev Med, 27*(3 Suppl.), 154-162.

Environmental Protection Agency. (2003). *Travel and environmental implications of school siting.* (No. EPA 231-R-03-004). Washington, DC: Author.

Feenstra, G. W. (1997). Local food systems and sustainable communities. *American Journal of Alternative Agriculture, 12*(1), 28-36.

Ferreira, I., van der Horst, K., Wendel-Vos, W., Kremers, S., van Lenthe, F. J., & Brug, J. (2007). Environmental correlates of physical activity in youth: A review and update. *Obesity Reviews, 8*(2), 129-154.

Fonseca, F. (2008, October 23). New Navajo law provides breastfeeding rights. *Associated Press*.

Hancox, R. J., Milne, B. J., & Poulton, R. (2004). Association between child and adolescent television viewing and adult health: A longitudinal birth cohort study. *Lancet, 364*(9430), 257-262.

Healthy Eating Active Communities. (2007). *Sites Baldwin Park*. Los Angeles, CA: Healthy Eating Active Communities.

Healthy Maine Partnerships. (2003). *Promoting trail development and use of safe community routes for walking and biking*. Augusta: Maine Department of Human Services.

Heath, G. W., Brownson, R. C., Kruger, J., Miles, R., Powell, K. E., & Ramsey, L. T. (2006). The effectiveness of urban design and land use and transport policies and practices to increase physical activity: A systematic review. *Journal of Physical and Activity and Health, 3*(suppl 1), S55-S76.

Holmes, G. (2009). Benefits of farm-to-school projects, healthy eating and physical activity for school children, *Field briefing testimony to the United States Senate Committee on Agriculture, Nutrition, and Forestry*. Atlanta, GA.

IOM. (2005). *Preventing childhood obesity: Health in the balance*. Washington, DC: The National Academies Press.

IOM. (2006). *Food marketing to children and youth: Threat or opportunity?* Washington, DC: The National Academies Press.

Joint Center for Political and Economic Studies and PolicyLink. (2004). *A place for healthier living: Improving access to physical activity and healthy foods*. Washington DC: Authors.

Kral, T. V., & Rolls, B. J. (2004). Energy density and portion size: Their independent and combined effects on energy intake. *Physiology and Behavior, 82*(1), 131-138.

Kubik, M. Y., Lytle, L. A., Hannan, P. J., Perry, C. L., & Story, M. (2003). The association of the school food environment with dietary behaviors of young adolescents. *Am J Public Health, 93*(7), 1168-1173.

Larson, N. I., Story, M. T., & Nelson, M. C. (2008). Neighborhood environments: Disparities in access to healthy foods in the U.S. *Am J Prev Med, 36*(1), 74-81.

LAUSD. (2002). *The Los Angeles Unified School District Healthy Beverage Motion*. Los Angeles, CA: LAUSD Business Services Division, Food Services.

League of American Bicyclists. (2005). *Bicycle friendly community program*. Washington, DC: League of American Bicyclists.

Live Well Colorado. (n.d.). The small steps for healthy leaps restaurant program. Retrieved June 9, 2009, from http://www.livewellcolorado.org/node/192

Local Government Commission Center for Livable Communities. (n.d.). *The economic benefits of walkable communities*. Sacramento, CA: Author.

Lockwood, I., & Stillings, T. (1998). *Traffic calming for crime reduction & neighborhood revitalization*. West Palm Beach, FL: City of West Palm Beach.

McCann, B. (2006). *Community design for healthy eating: How land use and transportation solutions can help*. Princeton, NJ: Robert Wood Johnson Foundation.

Mercedes Independent School District. (2005). *Mercedes Independent School District student nutrition/wellness plan*. Mercedes, TX: Author.

Metropolitan King County Council. (2006). *2004 King County comprehensive plan update*. Renton, WA: King County Department of Development and Environmental Services.

Mississippi Office of Healthy Schools. (2007). *Mississippi Healthy Students Act*. Jackson, MS: Author.

Montgomery County Blue Ribbon Panel on Pedestrian and Traffic Safety. (2002). *Setting safety in motion: Recommendations for creating walkable communities in Montgomery County, Maryland*. Bethesda, MD: Author.

Morland, K., Wing, S., & Diez Roux, A. (2002). The contextual effect of the local food environment on residents' diets: The atherosclerosis risk in communities study. *Am J Public Health, 92*(11), 1761-1767.

Morland, K., Wing, S., Diez Roux, A., & Poole, C. (2002). Neighborhood characteristics associated with the location of food stores and food service places. *Am J Prev Med, 22*(1), 23-29.

NASPE & AHA. (2006). *Shape of the nation report: Status of physical education in the USA*. Reston, VA: Authors.

National Association for Sport and Physical Education. (n.d.). NASPE STARS School: Equestrian Trails Elementary School. Retrieved May 18, 2009, from http://www.aahperd.org/Naspe/stars/schools_equestrian.html

National Center for Safe Routes to School. (2007). *Introduction to Safe Routes to School: The health, safety, and transportation nexus*. Chapel Hill, NC: Author.

New York City Department of Health and Mental Hygiene. (2006). Notice of adoption of amendments to Article 47 of the New York City health code. New York, NY: Author.

New York City Department of Health and Mental Hygiene. (2007). *Health department expands "Health Bucks" program to provide more coupons for fresh fruit and vegetables. Press release July 10, 2007.* New York, NY: New York City Department of Health and Mental Hygiene.

New York City Mayor's Office. (2008). Mayor Bloomberg and Shaquille O'Neal announce new food standards for city agencies, *Press Release*. New York: Author.

Ogden, C. L., Carroll, M. D., Curtin, L. R., McDowell, M. A., Tabak, C. J., & Flegal, K. M. (2006). Prevalence of overweight and obesity in the United States, 1999-2004. *Jama, 295*(13), 1549-1555.

Ogden, C. L., Carroll, M. D., & Flegal, K. M. (2008). High body mass index for age among U.S. children and adolescents, 2003-2006. *Jama, 299*(20), 2401-2405.

Oregon Transportation and Growth Management Program. (2005). *Planning for schools and liveable communities: The Oregon school siting handbook*. Salem, OR: Author.

Parker, T., & Arrington, G. B. (2002). *Statewide transit-oriented development study: Factors for success in California*. Sacramento, CA: California Department of Transportation.

PedNet Coalition. (2008). *PedNet: Pedestrian and pedaling network*. Columbia, MO: Author.

Perry, C. L., Bishop, D. B., Taylor, G., Murray, D. M., Mays, R. W., Dudovitz, B. S., et al. (1998). Changing fruit and vegetable consumption among children: The 5-a-Day Power Plus program in St. Paul, Minnesota. *Am J Public Health, 88*(4), 603-609.

PolicyLink & Bay Area Local Initiatives Support Corporation. (2008). *Grocery store attraction strategies: A resource guide for community activists and local governments*. Oakland, CA: Authors.

Public Transportation Partnership for Tomorrow. (2008). *Ten ways to enhance your community: Unleash the power of public transportation*. Washington, DC: Author.

Rolls, B. J., Roe, L. S., & Meengs, J. S. (2006). Reductions in portion size and energy density of foods are additive and lead to sustained decreases in energy intake. *Am J Clin Nutr, 83*(1), 11-17.

Saelens, B. E., Sallis, J. F., & Frank, L. D. (2003). Environmental correlates of walking and cycling: Findings from the transportation, urban design, and planning literatures. *Ann Behav Med, 25*(2), 80-91.

Seattle Public Schools. (2004). *Distribution and sales of competitive foods, board adopted procedure* (No. E 13.01). Seattle, WA: Author.

Shealy, K. R., Li, R., Benton-Davis, S., & Grummer-Strawn, L. (2005). *The CDC guide to breastfeeding interventions*. Atlanta, GA: Centers for Disease Control and Prevention.

Staunton, C. E., Hubsmith, D., & Kallins, W. (2003). Promoting safe walking and biking to school: the Marin County success story. *Am J Public Health, 93*(9), 1431-1434.

Strategic Alliance ENACT. (1998). Policy detail: Interim Land Use Policy. Retrieved May 6, 2009, from http://www.preventioninstitute.org/sa/policies/policy_detail.php?s_Search=Escondido&policyID=161

Strategic Alliance ENACT. (1999). Policy detail: Commercial Free Schools Act. Retrieved April 13, 2009, from http://www.preventioninstitute.org/sa/policies/search_results.php?s_Search=commercial+free+schools+act

Texas Department of State Health Services. (2008). *Tex Plate*. Austin, TX: Author.

University of Arkansas for Medical Sciences. (2008). *Year four evaluation: Arkansas Act 1220 of 2003 to Combat Childhood Obesity*. Little Rock, AR: Author.

Viner, R. M., & Cole, T. J. (2005). Television viewing in early childhood predicts adult body mass index. *J Pediatr, 147*(4), 429-435.

Weir, T. (2004, December 15). "New PE" objective: Get kids in shape. *USA Today*.

Winterfeld, A. P. (2007). *Healthy lifestyles, childhood obesity: Update of policy options and research*. Washington, DC: National Conference of State Legislatures.

Zaza, S., Briss, P. A., & Harris, K. W. (2005). *The guide to community preventive services: What works to promote health?* New York: Oxford University Press.

APPENDIX A:
PROJECT WORK GROUPS

Appendix A: Project Work Groups

Common Community Measures for Obesity Prevention Project Team

John Moore, PhD, RN, Katie Sobush, MS, MPH, Amy C. Lowry, MPA, Danielle Jackson, MPH, CDC Foundation; Susan Zaro, MPH, Dana Keener, PhD, Ken Goodman, MA, Jakub Kakietek, MPH, ICF Macro; Mark Thompson, MURP, Donald Gloo, MBA, International City/County Management Association; Erika Fulmer, MHA, Jeannette Renaud, PhD, Research Triangle Institute; Laura Kettel Khan, PhD, Division of Nutrition, Physical Activity, and Obesity, National Center for Chronic Disease Prevention and Health Promotion, CDC.

Funders Steering Committee

Celeste Torio, PhD, Laura Leviton, PhD, Robert Wood Johnson Foundation; Loel Solomon, MPH, Kaiser Permanente; Linda Jo Doctor, MPH, W. K. Kellogg Foundation; Mary Gray, RD, U.S. Department of Agriculture; Robert Kuczmarski, PhD, Amy Yaroch, PhD, National Institutes of Health.

CDC Technical Advisors

William Dietz, MD, PhD, Deborah Galuska, PhD, Casey Hannan, MPH, Jude McDivitt, PhD, Division of Nutrition, Physical Activity, and Obesity, National Center for Chronic Disease Prevention and Health Promotion; Sam Posner, PhD, Office of the Director, National Center for Chronic Disease Prevention and Health Promotion, CDC.

Select Panelists

Frances Butterfoss, PhD, Eastern Virginia Medical School, Division of Behavioral Research & Community Health; Laura Brennen, PhD, Transtria LLC; Allen Cheadle, PhD, University of Washington, Health Promotion Research Center; John Cook, PhD, Boston University, School of Medicine, Department of Pediatrics; Reid Ewing, PhD, University of Maryland; Brian Flay, PhD, Oregon State University, College of Health & Human Sciences; Penny Gordon-Larsen, PhD, University of North Carolina at Chapel Hill, Department of Nutrition, Schools of Public Health and Medicine, Michael Hamm, PhD, Michigan State University, Department of Food Science & Human Nutrition, Jeffrey Harris, DrPH, MPH, RD, LDN, Westchester University, Nutrition & Dietetics Program; Laurie LaChance, PhD, University of Michigan, School of Public Health; Leslie Lytle, PhD, University of Minnesota, Division of Epidemiology & Community Health; Brian Saelens, PhD, University of Washington, Pediatrics; James Sallis, PhD, San Diego State University, Department of Psychology; Sarah Samuels, DrPH, Samuels & Associates; Gail Woodward-Lopez, MPH, University of California–Berkeley, Center for Weight and Health

CDC Workgroup and Internal Content Area Experts

Heidi Blanck, PhD, Leigh Ramsey Buchanan, PhD, David Dennison, MPH, Diane Dunet, PhD, Jackie Epping, PhD, Cathleen Gillespie, MS, Alison Heintz, Claire Heiser, MPH, Joel Kimmons, PhD, Sarah Kuester, MS, Kimberly Lane, PhD, RD, Carol MacGowan, MPH, Latetia Moore, PhD, Christopher Reinold, MPH, Candace Rutt, PhD, Tom Schmid, PhD, Jenna Seymour, PhD, Andrea Sharma, PhD, MPH, Katherine Shealy, MPH, Bettylou Sherry, PhD, Diane Thompson, MPH, Edward Weiss, MD, Holly Wethington, PhD, Division of Nutrition, Physical Activity, and Obesity; Sarah Lee, PhD, Terry O'Toole, MDiv, PhD, Seraphine Pitt-Barnes, PhD, Leah Robin, PhD, Division of Adolescent and School Health; Indu Ahluwalia, PhD, Alyssa Easton, PhD, Marilyn Metzler, RN, Fred Ramsey, MS Michael Sells, MSPH, CHES, Alexandria Stewart, Division of Adult and Community Health; Ralph Coates, PhD, Temeika Fairley, PhD, Staci Lofton, MPH, Phyllis Rochester, PhD, Division of Cancer Prevention and Control; Ann Albright, PhD, RD Carmen Harris, MPH, Qaiser Mukhtar, PhD, Dawn Satterfield, PhD, Division of Diabetes Translation; Michael Schooley, MPH, Division of Heart Disease and Stroke Prevention; Connie Bish, PhD, Shin Kim, MPH, Division of Reproductive Health; Nicole Kuiper, MPH, Natalie Whitney, MPH, Office on Smoking and Health, National Center for Chronic Disease Prevention and Health Promotion; Sarah Heaton, MPH, Susan Hobson, Dee Merriam, MLA, Heather Morrow-Almeida, MPH, Division of Environmental and Emergency Health Services; Anjana Banerjee, MPH, Division of Environmental Hazards and Health Effects, National Center for Injury Prevention and Control; Laurie Beck, MPH, Division of Unintentional Injury Prevention; Joanne Klevens, PhD, Division of Violence Prevention, National Center for Environmental Health, CDC.

Measurement Experts

Allen Cheadle, PhD, University of Washington, Health Promotion Research Center; Brian Flay, PhD, Oregon State University, College of Health and Human Sciences; Tom Holland, Nish Keshav, MPA, MA, Center for Performance Measurement, International City/County Management Association; Michael Schooley, MPH, Division of Heart Disease and Stroke Prevention, National Center for Chronic Disease Prevention and Health Promotion, Sue Lin Yee, MPH, Office of the Director, CDC.

Local Government Experts

Wes Hare, MS, City Manager, City of Albany, Oregon; Thomas Forslund, MPA, City Manager, City of Casper, Wyoming; Peggy Merriss, MPA, City Manager, City of Decatur, Georgia; Amanda Thompson, MPA, Planning Director, City of Decatur, Georgia; David Ramsey, City Manager, City of Kirkland, Washington; Bonnie Svrcek, MPA, Deputy City Manager, City of Lynchburg, Virginia; Rick Freas, MPA, Deputy Budget and Research Director, City of Phoenix, Arizona.

Pilot Test Communities

City of Albany, OR; City of Arlington, TX; City of Bridgeport, CT; City of Casper, WY; Chesterfield County, VA; City of Coral Springs, FL; City of Decatur, GA; City of Eugene, OR; Fairfax County, VA; City of Fort Collins, CO; City of Grain Valley, MO; City of Highland Park, IL; City of Lynchburg, VA; City of North Las Vegas, NV; City of Oklahoma City, OK; Santa Barbara County, CA; City of Sioux Falls, SD; Borough of State College, PA; City of Vancouver, WA; City of Woodbury, MN

Appendix B:
Terms Used in This Manual

Appendix B: Terms Used in This Manual

Bike lanes: As defined by the American Association of State Highway and Transportation Officials, portions of a roadway that have been designated by striping, signing, and pavement markings for the preferential or exclusive use of bicyclists.

Bike routes: Cycling routes on roads shared with motorized vehicles or on specially marked sidewalks.

Coalition: A group of persons representing diverse public- or private-sector organizations or constituencies working together to achieve a shared goal through coordinated use of resources, leadership, and action.

Competitive foods and beverages: All foods and beverages served or sold in schools that are not part of Federal school meal programs, including "à la carte" items sold in cafeterias and items sold in vending machines. As defined by the Institute of Medicine (2005), competitive foods and beverages typically are lower in nutritional quality than those offered by school meal programs.

Complete streets: As defined by the National Complete Streets Coalition (http://www.completestreets.org), streets that are designed and operated to enable safe access along and across the street for all users, including pedestrians, bicyclists, motorists, and transit riders of all ages and abilities.

Eating occasion: A single meal or snack.

Energy density: The number of calories per gram in weight.

Environmental change: An alteration or change to physical, social, or economic environments designed to influence people's practices and behaviors.

Farm stand: Multiple and single vendors that are not part of a licensed farmers market.

Farmer-day: Any part of a calendar day spent by a farmer (vendor) at a farmers market (excluding craft vendors and prepared food vendors). The total number of annual farmer-days for a given farmers market is based on the number of days that the farmers market is open in a year multiplied by the number of farm vendors at the market on a given day.

Full-service grocery store: A medium to large food retail store that sells a variety of food products, including some perishable items and general merchandise.

Healthier foods and beverages: As defined by Institute of Medicine (2005), foods and beverages with low energy density and low content of calories, sugar, fat, and sodium.

Largest school district within a local jurisdiction: The school district that serves the largest number of students within a local jurisdiction.

Less healthy foods and beverages: As defined by Institute of Medicine (2005), foods and beverages with a high content of calories, sugar, fat, and sodium, and low content of nutrients, including protein, vitamins A and C, niacin, riboflavin, thiamin, calcium, and iron.

Local government facilities: Facilities owned, leased, or operated by a local government (including facilities that might be owned or leased by a local government but operated by contracted employees). For the purposes of this project, and according to the definition established by ICMA, local government facilities might include facilities in the following categories:

- **24-hour "dormitory-type" facilities:** facilities that generally are in operation 24 hours per day, 7 days per week, such as firehouses (and their equipment bays), women's shelters, men's shelters, and group housing facilities for children, seniors, and physically or mentally challenged persons, not including regular public housing;

- **administrative/office facilities:** general office buildings, court buildings, data processing facilities, sheriff's offices (including detention facilities), 911 centers, social service intake centers, day care/preschool facilities, historical buildings, and other related facilities;

- **detention facilities:** jails, adult detention centers, juvenile detention centers, and related facilities;

- **health care facilities:** hospitals, clinics, morgues, and related facilities;

- **recreation/community center facilities:** senior centers, community centers, gymnasiums, public parks and fields, and other similar recreation centers, including concession stands located at these facilities; and

- **other facilities:** water treatment plants, airports, schools, and all other facilities that do not explicitly fall into the categories listed above.

Low energy dense foods and beverages: Foods and beverages with a low calorie-per-gram ratio. Foods with a high water and fiber content are low in energy density, such as fruits, vegetables, and broth-based soups and stews.

Measure: For the purpose of this project, a measure is defined as a single data element that can be collected through an objective assessment of the physical or policy environment and used to quantify without bias an obesity prevention strategy.

Mixed-use development: Zoning that combines residential land use with one or more of the following types of land use: commercial, industrial, or other public use.

Network distance: Shortest distance between two locations by way of the public street network.

Nonmotorized transportation: Any form of transportation that does not involve the use of a motorized vehicle, such as walking and biking.

Nutrition standards: Criteria that determine which foods and beverages may be offered in a particular setting (e.g., schools or local government facilities). Nutrition standards may be defined locally or adopted from national standards.

Partnership: A business-like arrangement that might involve two or more partner organizations.

Policy: Laws, regulations, rules, protocols, and procedures designed to guide or influence behavior. Policies can be either legislative or organizational in nature.

Portion size: The amount of a single food item served in a single eating occasion (e.g., a meal or a snack). Portion size is the amount (e.g., weight, caloric content, or volume) of food offered to a person in a restaurant, the amount in the packaging of prepared foods, or the amount a person chooses to put on his or her plate. One portion of food might contain several USDA food servings.

Pricing strategies: Intentional adjustment to the unit cost of an item (e.g., offering a discount on a food item, selling a food item at a lower profit margin, or banning a surcharge on a food item).

Public recreation facility: Facility listed in the local jurisdiction's facility inventory that has at least one amenity that promotes physical activity (e.g., walking/hiking trail, bicycle trail, or open play field/play area).

Public recreation facility entrance: The point of entry to a facility that permits recreation. For the purposes of this project, geographic information system (GIS) coordinates of the entrance to a recreational facility or the street address of the facility.

Public service venue: Facilities and settings open to the public that are managed under the authority of government entities (e.g., schools, child care centers, community recreational facilities, city and county buildings, prisons, and juvenile detention centers).

Public transit stop: Point of entrance to a local jurisdiction's transportation and public street network, such as bus stops, light rail stops, and subway stations.

School siting: The process of locating schools and school facilities.

Screen (viewing) time: Time spent watching television, playing video games, and engaging in noneducational computer activities.

Shared-use paths: As defined by the American Association of State Highway and Transportation Officials, bikeways used by cyclists, pedestrians, skaters, wheelchair users, joggers, and other nonmotorized users that are physically separated from motorized vehicular traffic by an open space or barrier and within either the highway right-of-way or an independent right-of-way.

Sidewalk network: An interconnected system of paved walkways designated for pedestrian use, usually located beside a street or roadway.

Street network: A system of interconnecting streets and intersections for a given area.

Sugar-sweetened beverages: Beverages that contain added caloric sweeteners, primarily sucrose derived from cane, beets, and corn (high-fructose corn syrup), including non-diet carbonated soft drinks, flavored milks, fruit drinks, teas, and sports drinks.

Supermarket: A large, corporate-owned food store with annual sales of at least $2 million.

Underserved census tract: Within metropolitan areas, a census tract that is characterized by one of the following criteria: (i) a median income at or below 120% of the median income of the metropolitan area and a minority population of 30% or greater; or (ii) a median income at or below 90% of median income of the metropolitan area. In rural, nonmetropolitan areas, the following criteria should be used instead: (i) a median income at or below 120% of the greater of the State nonmetropolitan median income or the nationwide nonmetropolitan median income and a minority population of 30% or greater; or (ii) a median income at or below 95% of the greater of the State nonmetropolitan median income or nationwide nonmetropolitan median income (Department of Housing and Urban Development, 1995).

Violent crime: A legal offense that involves force or threat of force. According to the Federal Bureau of Investigation's Uniform Crime Reporting (UCR) Program, violent crime includes murder, forcible rape, robbery, and aggravated assault <http://www.fbi.gov/ucr/cius2007/offenses/violent_crime/index.html>.

APPENDIX C:
USEFUL CONTACTS FOR DATA COLLECTION

Appendix C: Useful Contacts for Data Collection

Association of State and Territorial Public Health Nutrition Directors (ASTPHND)
<http://www.astphnd.org>

ASTPHND Designees and Fruit & Vegetable Nutrition Coordinators
<http://www.astphnd.org/members_directory.php?sid=123be3&key_words_array%5B%5D=3&origin=side_menu%20>

Coordinated School Health Programs Funded by the Division of Adolescence and School Health
<http://www.cdc.gov/healthyYouth/partners/funded/cshp.htm>

National Society of Physical Activity Practitioners in Public Health (NSPAPPH)
<http://www.nspapph.org/>

NSPAPPH State Physical Activity Coordinators
<http://www.nspapph.org/index.php?option=com_mtree&Itemid=45%20>

State Programs Funded by the Division of Nutrition, Physical Activity, and Obesity
<http://www.cdc.gov/nccdphp/dnpa/obesity/state_programs/funded_states/index.htm>

www.ingramcontent.com/pod-product-compliance
Lightning Source LLC
Chambersburg PA
CBHW081733170526
45167CB00009B/3803